Secrets of the Obvious:

A Guide for Balanced Living

by Harry Cohen, Ph.D.

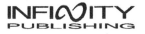
INFINITY
PUBLISHING

Copyright © 2002 by Harry David Cohen, Ph.D.

ISBN 0-7414-1369-8

Published by:

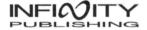

INFINITY PUBLISHING
1094 New DeHaven Street, Suite 100
West Conshohocken, PA 19428-2713
Toll-free (877) BUY BOOK
Local Phone (610) 941-9999
Fax (610) 941-9959
Info@buybooksontheweb.com
www.buybooksontheweb.com

Printed in the United States of America

Published November 2010

Contents

Chapter 1   Balance and Performance......1

The Question.. 2

Out of Balance.. 5

What I'm *Not* Saying.. 8

The Big Seven 11

In Balance..12

Performance...14

Gender and Age..15

Secrets of the Obvious 17

Chapter 2   Put Gas in Your Tank 19

Supply and Demand..21

Four Options 22

    1. Reduce External Demand 22

    2. Reduce Internal Demand......................30

    3. Increase External Supply.....................32

    4. Increase Internal Supply 35

Secrets of the Obvious 39

Chapter 3   Progress, Not Perfection......41

Lighten Up! 43

The Gap..45

The Key to Misery 47

The Secret...49

Effort and Grace 51

Secrets of the Obvious 55

Chapter 4 Physical Health 57

Sleep *61*

Water *63*

Smoking *66*

Nutrition *66*

Caffeine *71*

Alcohol *73*

Exercise *73*

Relaxation *80*

Health Checkups *81*

Secrets of the Obvious *83*

Chapter 5 Psychological Health 85

Pay Attention *87*

Being Stupid *89*

In Perspective *94*

Your Sense of Humor *97*

Putting Yourself Down *101*

Take Charge of Your Emotions *106*

Positive Self-Talk *109*

Secrets of the Obvious *112*

Chapter 6 Social Health 113

Good Company *116*

Toxic People *119*

Jerks *122*

Listening *123*

A Third Place *125*

Integrity *126*

Most Important Words *126*

What Goes Around *133*

Secrets of the Obvious *134*

Chapter 7 Health at Work 135

Love It or Leave It *136*

Your Unique Abilities *140*

Good at Something *144*

Your Brand *147*

Problems and Challenges *151*

Meaning in Your Work *154*

A Culture of Excellence *157*

Get Organized *160*

Make Your Own Lunch *162*

Secrets of the Obvious *164*

Chapter 8 Family Health 165

Marriage *166*

Kids *173*

Parents *188*

Secrets of the Obvious *192*

Chapter 9 Financial Health 193

Saving *194*

Waste and Value *196*

Investing *200*

Debt *202*

Buying Smart: The Law of Tuna Fish and Toilet Paper. 205

Speculation 207

Giving It Away 209

Your Money or Your Life 210

Secrets of the Obvious 214

Chapter 10 Spiritual Health 215

Be a Seeker 217

Karma and Dharma 222

Meditate or Pray 226

Leave a Legacy 230

Secrets of the Obvious 233

Chapter 11 Obviously, Not the End 235

Desiderata 236

Secrets on the Web 239

About the Author 239

Acknowledgements

There are so many people who enabled me to write this book, that I was struggling to figure out how to adequately thank them all. Several people — half kiddingly — said that it didn't matter *who* I acknowledged as long as I thanked *them*. This confirmed my fear that naming names would eventually get me into hot water with someone I neglected to mention.

The book is also filled with anecdotes about people who have taught me or influenced me in some way. In fact, when I've given the draft to friends and colleagues, they've often said something like, "I enjoyed it a great deal, but I would have liked to see a few more stories about me." Be that as it may, I do want to thank my family, my friends, and my colleagues. They have taught me and given me so much, that it is impossible to appropriately express my gratitude. A "no-names mentioned" but very heartfelt "thank you" will have to do for now.

For Herman and Millicent,
who taught me the meaning of balance

Why This Book?

In my twenty years of speaking to groups in corporations and counseling individuals in my private practice, there is one principle that has never changed: Every single person on one level or another longs for a better life.

"Better" means different things to different people at different times, of course. Yet every time I speak about the importance of living a better life by living a more *balanced* life, people can relate. It's clear that they crave help in balancing the multiple demands and pressures of life in a simple way that allows them to be both successful and fulfilled. People can certainly be materially successful but also incredibly unfulfilled. I believe, however, that it doesn't have to be an "either-or" proposition. We can be both. It's not rocket science, and most people are familiar with what I have to say. Surprisingly, though, when I present these concepts in a lecture, they often act as if they were hearing them for the first time.

Most important for me, however, is that as I practice what I preach more consistently, my life is more balanced and I'm more successful and fulfilled. My experience as a student, psychologist, consultant, speaker, husband, father, friend, son, brother and seeker has taught me that it works. So one reason I'm writing this book is that these ideas have made a profound difference in my own life, helping me and other people in hundreds of ways that I'll tell you about in the following pages. Plus, there's another reason: **Mediocrity is a drag. It's just more fun to raise the bar.**

I'm also writing this book for my father, Herman Cohen. My Dad died in December of 1995, and I miss him even more as time passes. He taught me so much about how to live a decent life that I would love to share some of his wisdom. Who we become as people has a lot to do with the parents we were given, the teachers in our lives, the friends we surround ourselves with, and the choices we make in our very short lives. I wish my father were alive today. In some ways he modeled what I'm talking about. He was by no means perfect in all of these areas, but he did keep them all in perspective up until his death. I suppose one legacy he left was the simple message of this book: **Take care of the basics.**

My Dad also taught me a lot about making choices, and the consequences of those choices. When I was a teenager he put a huge sign in my bedroom that read, "Procrastination is the thief of time."

I had been putting off writing this book for years for a million reasons:

> *I have to wait until my dissertation is done... When the twins get a little older... When the Ford project is up and running... When we finish building the new house... When I'm not traveling so much...*

Blah! Blah! Blah! It's time. This book is for you, Herm. Thank you. In the immortal words of Yul Brynner in *The Ten Commandments*, "So let it be written, so let it be done."

– Harry Cohen, Ann Arbor, Michigan, July 2002

Chapter 1

Balance and Performance

Greg has been a friend for years. As a social worker and a therapist, he's a smart man and a wise man. He's also a smoker — two packs a day for over 27 years. He's now in his early 50s.

His wife, Linda, suffers from one of those nasty, chronic, non-specific, undiagnosable diseases. She has been suffering from it for years, and of course Greg is also suffering as he watches her steady deterioration and possible death.

Greg has responded to the enormous strain in his life in a number of ways: He's thrown himself into his work, took up biking, and stopped his caffeine intake after noon — somehow, bright as he is, Greg never paid much attention to the caffeine-sleep connection.

In other words, Greg did a lot of things to restore a healthy balance in his life, and doing so enhanced his performance as a husband, as a professional, and as a caring human being.

But he continued to smoke.

1

Then he had what the doctors called "a heart event" — not a heart attack, but serious. The doctors found that one of his coronary arteries was 100% blocked, another 91% blocked. "You are lucky to be alive," his physician told him. "You should have had a heart attack." After he was taken to the hospital and they put a stent in one of his arteries, he had a lot of time to reflect. That was Greg's wake-up call.

Greg is now biking over 100 miles a week and is steadily losing weight. He even quit smoking — cold turkey. He knows it won't be easy to regain his balance — he's a human being like the rest of us — but he's finally moving in the right direction.

The Question

Here's my question: **Why must it take the impending death of a loved one, or your own near-death experience, to get you to do what you already know you should be doing?**

Greg is a very intelligent man, and he responded to Linda's illness by doing many of the things I advocate in this book. He looked after his physical health, getting more exercise and keeping a lid on his drinking and caffeine. He balanced his energy for work and family, and he connected with his friends. He rediscovered the spiritual perspective in his life.

That was great, but it was not enough. It took a glimpse of his own death to make Greg really "get it." And by that time, he had to go to extremes — cold turkey nicotine withdrawal and 100+ miles per week on his bike — to restore his life to balance. My point is this: **Had he been balancing the different areas of his life better in the first place, he would not have had such a close call.**

Of course, we don't know if his early action would have had any impact on Linda's health problems. Probably not. But Greg's doctor is right — he's a lucky man. He has taken advantage of that luck to turn his life around. But isn't it better to turn it around before the crisis hits so that we will be solidly on our feet, ready to perform in the often unpredictable ways life demands of us? Especially if it involves remembering to do some of the things that we probably already know we should be doing. Secrets of the Obvious.

> *Recently, I was out for a jog and I ran into a guy, a total stranger, who had some sort of device attached to his chest. I struck up a conversation with him, and he told me it was a heart monitor. I asked him why he was wearing it. "I had a heart attack two years ago," he explained, "and it changed my life." Why should it take a heart attack for him to change? We are the species with the big brains. We know the consequences of our actions. We can read*

*about heart attacks and how to prevent
them without having one of our own.*

Greg's situation is not unusual, though its seriousness
may be. The specific details, of course, will vary. But lots
of people find their lives out of balance today, and a
crisis of one kind or another is eventually just around the
corner. It may not be life-threatening as in the case of
Greg and Linda, but it will be something — something at
work, something in the family, something in your own
health or the health of a loved one. Something that will
require us to perform at our highest levels. **Crises
happen.** Stuff happens. You know what I mean. **There
is no way we can go through life and not be tested
by life events.** So how can we be prepared to deal with
whatever comes our way — and maybe even save our
life? By "deal with" I really mean handle with grace and
equanimity, not with teeth clenched, gasping for air. The
goal is to move through challenges without freaking out.
**When crises do happen, the goal is not to merely
survive, but to thrive.**

I'm not simply trying to warn you about stress and to
suggest stress management techniques, though many
business groups I have talked with find what I have to
say very useful in dealing with the accelerating pressures
in the competitive corporate world. But leading a
balanced life is the way to improve your performance in
all areas of your life — on the job, but also as a husband
or wife, as a father or mother, son or daughter, or friend.
Leading a balanced life will make you a better person. A
more effective person. A higher performing person. A
more satisfied person. A happier person. A more fulfilled

4

person. A person who can handle adversity and tragedy with grace. This is true, I believe, whether you are facing the stress of a crisis or dealing with the routine demands of your life. **Performance matters.**

Why do some people juggle multiple demands and responsibilities with grace, while other people facing the exact same circumstances wither and fold? There is a reason — and it's not just bad luck. In fact, luck has nothing to do with it. **Balance matters.**

Out of Balance

In my give and take with large audiences and with private patients, it is rare that I come across people who feel that their lives are in a good balance. How do our lives get so out of balance? I suppose the simplest answer is the best one: because there is no guarantee that the stuff life sends your way will leave you in good balance. You know what it's like — a sudden accident or illness, a letter about an IRS audit, a pregnant daughter, a phone call from a friend in crisis, a note that your company is being downsized. Stuff like that can knock you flat on your back. Given all that, it's perfectly normal to find that you have to work at it to keep yourself — your life — in balance. **The real question is not why our lives are so often out of balance, but rather, how can we keep them in better balance?**

I say "in better balance" because balance exists on a continuum. You are not either in or out of balance but usually somewhere in between, and moving in one direction or the other. It works the same as the continuum between being slightly irritated and clinically depressed, or between a bit out of shape and morbidly obese. Nobody can perfectly cultivate and balance *everything*, and trying to be perfect will be frustrating. In much the same way: **Nobody's life is stress-free until the moment of death.**

But we can nudge ourselves into better balance. So when I refer to living "a balanced life," I really mean a life that is in better balance — more toward the healthy side of the continuum.

By living in balance I also mean not going so overboard on one thing that you neglect all others. The easy target here is the workaholic who neglects his family and probably his physical health and a few other important aspects of his life along the way. But others can be equally imbalanced in other directions. Think of a person who devotes so much time to family that she lets her social relationships outside of her family atrophy, and possibly her physical and psychological health at the same time. Greg had to work energetically to keep his preoccupation with his wife's tragic illness from destroying his life in the process. Preoccupation with family is a frequent complaint of stay-at-home mothers and fathers, or people who find themselves in caretaker roles with family members. Others can be so imbalanced toward financial health that they never take a vacation with their families and won't join a gym — no time, too expensive. Such people may be so focused on financial health that their work health actually suffers, for they may be working exclusively for the money, taking no joy in what they are doing and therefore doing it less well.

But the imbalance can occur without all the weight being thrown on one area of your life. Often something important to us simply gets neglected. Not just neglected once in a while, or for short periods of time when you are unusually busy with something else, but chronically or habitually neglected. You just don't do any family stuff — that's your wife's department, so she's the one who calls your mom on Mother's Day. Or, you are great with your family and your job, you exercise and save regularly, but you do all this because you are driven by guilt: You will go to Hell if you don't lead a Perfectly Responsible Life. Or, you neglect your friendships because you're so busy with work and family. Or, you're so busy making money that you don't take stock to see how you're spending it or investing it. **Getting out of shape didn't just happen.**

The point is, that if we completely neglect one or two areas of our lives, it will eventually nail us or, at best, slow us down. **You can drive your car with only a few of the lug nuts tightened, but not very far and not very fast.**

Some of us can become so obsessed with a source of immediate pressure that we totally lose perspective on our lives. Other people find themselves dashing about from one source of stress to another, so pretty soon all they are aware of is this dashing about and not the things — let's call them "your life" — that exist between dashes. Our body keeps score when this happens.

I speak for a living so it's not real good when I get a sore throat and sound like a croaking frog in front of 150 people. During cold and flu season I'm particularly vulnerable to catching a cold and losing my voice. The reason I do is always the same: I run myself down from working too hard, not getting enough sleep, not eating right, and worrying about things I can't control. The pattern usually goes like this: I stop exercising for a few days, stay up until midnight a couple of nights, have a fight with someone at work, and count the days until the weekend. Boom! The next thing I know, I have that little tickle in the back of my throat. **I finally figured out that if I take a red-eye back from California, I pay for it. The body always keeps score.**

Lewis Thomas described his wonder at the mysteries of the central nervous system by saying that our brains are smarter than we are. Well, in some ways our bodies are smarter than we are, too.

What I'm Not Saying

Here's another way to look at the situation: You hear a lot of talk these days about finding "a proper balance between work and life." Can you see how that statement of a goal has a built-in problem? That's like saying that your diet should include a proper balance of apples and fruit. Your work is *part of* your life, not something external to your life that you can balance against it. Because of this, you need to make sure that you see your work in the context of the various other aspects of your life. The main idea underlying this book is that attending to these different aspects will make you more high-performing and lead you to feelings of fulfillment and success.

It may help if you can see something else I am not saying. I'm not saying that if only you worked on One Really Important Thing — if only you became a vegetarian, or practiced daily meditation, or quit drinking, or joined the wine-tasting club, or forgave your parents, or got in touch with your inner child, or got in touch with your inner adult, or beat a drum with the guys in the woods, etc. — then your life would be fulfilled and successful. Nonsense — for most of us — though if any of that stuff works for you, well good, then do it. No, the model I have in mind, to say it again, is one based on balance. There are seven rather obvious but, nonetheless, very important areas in our lives. Keep them in some sort of balance by paying attention, in your own way, to each of them, and your life will get better. That sense of balance feels good, and it's productive on a number of fronts. That sense of balance may be **a means to success**, and in fact, it may even **be success.**

> *My friend Doug is a successful attorney in private practice. He taught himself to litigate and has become a full partner in his law firm. He has a great marriage right now and two young children. One of his kids is a special needs child who requires a full-time aide at school. The little boy's problems are complex and challenging, and are compounded by a severe food allergy. There is an epinephrine pen*

9

wherever he goes. You can imagine the challenge of being a good father, husband and provider, while maintaining some semblance of a life.

Doug has been dealing with a lot for the past couple of years and has let his body get to the point where he has perfected the "before" picture in these weight loss testimonial shots. He hates the way he looks. He feels exhausted most of the time, and his back is frequently sore from carrying the load in his gut. He just recently decided it was time to get in shape. He's been working out, drinking tons of water, and losing weight. For the first time in years, he told me, his back isn't hurting. Here's a guy who didn't have to have a heart attack to get it together.

Here's yet another thing I'm not saying: Deal with stress, and your life will come into balance. What I'm saying is the reverse of that: **Bring your life into balance, and you will be able to deal with stress more effectively.**

Look, nobody says, "Hey, I'm managing my stress now — when I'm done, I'll get back to my life." It obviously doesn't work that way. You are living your life right now. Your life **is** stress. What I'm saying is that if you manage your life better, then you will be managing the stress better.

Of course, there's always the possibility that if we just wait, balance will return on its own. Yes, that's exactly the same way that the Internal Revenue Service goes away when we ignore filing a tax return. And our marriage will get so much more satisfying just from being together. And I'm sure the weight will come off eventually. Buying lottery tickets is an excellent means of retirement planning. I'll get some friends when I retire and have more time. **Our balance is not likely to return, or even be maintained, on its own, without effort.**

If we get started now, we won't have to work at it as hard as Greg does, or have to have some horrible crisis knock us for a loop. The truth is that we have already started; the challenge is to do it consciously.

The Big Seven

When I talk about balance, what I mean is balancing what I call the "seven areas of healthy living." **Pay attention to each of them.** Take some sort of brief, but regular, inventory so we know we aren't neglecting any of these crucial aspects of human success and meaning.

1. **Physical**
2. **Psychological**
3. **Social**
4. **Work**
5. **Family**
6. **Financial**
7. **Spiritual**

These are the elements that you should work to keep in better balance. You probably know this already. If you are like most people, you need reminding of the obvious — just because we're human.

In Balance

When I was young and stupid I thought it intelligent and prudent not to fill the gas tank of my car. So I'd go and put just a couple of dollar's worth in at a time, reasoning that if I did that, I'd be spending less on gas and therefore saving money.

Well, now I know better. I realize that it pays to have plenty of gas in your tank so you won't run out during that surprisingly long stretch between stops, or you won't have to pull over and refill when you are in a hurry to get your kid to the hospital or yourself to the job interview or meeting you are going to be late for. Of course, I'm not really talking about gas here.

There are other ways to describe what I mean. **Living a balanced and high-performing life means having more tools in your toolbox.**

Comparing the balanced life to having gas in your tank suggests having enough energy or stamina to deal with the demanding situations — both the routine ones and the crises — at work, at home, on the road, on the telephone, or wherever. Having more tools in your toolbox suggests that you have a greater repertoire of skills and resources available to deal with the incredible

12

variety of difficult situations you will confront. Some of them will require prayer, meditation or whatever way you use to check in with your deepest values and beliefs. Others will require the ability to go to family members for love and support, or to give them love and support. Most of them will require sufficient physical health to keep your mind fresh, your spirits up. Most will also require self-discipline, knowing your limitations, a sense of humor, or grit. In other words, you probably can't count on one thing to get you through. A sense of humor does not solve everything; no more than does the ability to run a marathon. Unfortunately, for most people, neither does prayer, or having lots of good friends. It helps to have a variety of tools in your toolbox. **The seven areas of healthy living will help you perform better because you will have more energy and more internal and external resources.**

On occasion I have also described what I mean in terms of having more bullets in your gun. But the more I think about it, the less I like that analogy. The idea is not to shoot and kill the challenges in your life, but to dance with them and grow through the process. Think of it in terms of those difficult problems that your high school math teacher made you do as homework. The point is not that you solve the problem, but that the problem solves you: The process of dealing with the problem forces you to do a new kind of thinking, expanding your mind, changing yourself. In the same way, I don't think the point of your life is to destroy the larger problems you encounter. Resolve them, yes — but in doing so, strengthen the skills you use in the process.

13

Performance

The relationship between balance and performance should be obvious, but let me state a few of those obvious points. For most of us, life is not just the high jump or the 100-meter dash. It's more like a decathlon — ten events — and then throw in diaper changing, tire changing and getting told off by your boss. **While certain jobs might be for specialists, your life is not.**

On your job, you might be able to concentrate your time and energy on what you are good at and, to some extent, you might be able to do that at home. But the Big Picture says that you will be required to use a wide repertoire of skills and resources. You are going to be asked to perform — as a parent, or a husband, daughter, friend, colleague and leader, as a citizen of your community or the planet. To a large extent, you don't get to choose among these roles.

So we have to balance the different roles we will be asked to perform in our lives. What happens when you do this is that you achieve an internal balance as well. You probably know someone who has achieved that internal sense of balance — someone who seems to have it together, who in an unflustered way can shift gears from one role to another. These people seem to be deeply resourceful, combining internal strengths of mind, body and spirit along with connections to family, friends and community to which they give their time and attention, but from which they can also draw strength and wisdom when their circumstances require it. They

14

are able to perform at such high levels because of the breadth and depth of the resources they have available. Chances are, they have put time and energy into creating that balanced portfolio of strengths. **It's not an accident that these people are balanced. They do things to be that way.**

You may have had periods in your life when you felt that resourceful, that well-balanced. It feels good to be performing on all cylinders. And you know what? It feels good to be in the company of such a person — to be married to one, to work for or with one, to have one for a friend. Their level of balance and performance brings out the best in people around them. They are interesting. They are cool. They are inspiring.

Maintaining your strengths in all seven areas of healthy living gives you flexibility and balance in all the roles you will be asked to perform. It's a bit like cross-training, where the workouts prepare you for a variety of challenges.

Gender and Age

Gender and age don't matter here. Whatever your situation is, it just makes sense to keep these seven different areas of your life in a healthy balance. **All of us need balance.**

Similarly, it's true that at different stages of our lives we may have different priorities, and it's in a sense natural or developmental to shift from one priority to the next. When we have small children, it makes sense that family will become more of a priority. When we are starting a new job, work will be more important. When we are cruising for a mate, our physical health — or at least our appearance — will be more important. And when we are getting old and ready to die, our life may take a turn for the spiritual. Yes, these life-stages may exercise a certain amount of control over the way we prioritize among the seven areas of healthy living. But isn't that all the more reason to remind ourselves to bring them into balance? It's also true that life doesn't make it easy for us by sorting its challenges into neat chronological stages. You may be having your first baby at the same time that you are trying to impress that first boss with your dedication to the company. If it were all neat and simple, nobody would need a book like this one.

I'm not talking about perfect balance, just an improved balance: You can probably do better than you are doing now. The result will be higher performance, however you choose to measure it.

Secrets of the Obvious

- It should not take a near-death experience to remind us to take better care of ourselves

- Pay attention to the seven areas of healthy living: physical, psychological, social, work, family, financial and spiritual

- A balanced and healthy life leads to improved performance

- Balanced living requires effort

- Get started now. It will make a difference

Chapter 2

Put Gas in Your Tank

Dave, a man I know, was having a rough day. That afternoon he had sat in on a two-hour meeting with his son and his son's divorce attorney. The topic: the likelihood of a custody dispute. Dave's son was clearly confused and distressed, and it spilled over to Dave, who was trying to put up a calm and reassuring front. Later in the day he picked up his car from the garage, where he learned that a minor repair had swollen into a major $1,500 calamity, and then on the way home he discovered that the problem had not been fixed.

That evening, while watching television with his wife, the bottom dropped out. They were watching a program about child abuse, and somehow that triggered a flood of tears caused by the stresses of the day. Dave's wife, not knowing the reason for her husband's breakdown, slid over on the couch and held him in her arms. He blurted out a few words about why he was so upset, and she quietly reassured him: "How great that you are there for your son (her stepson). You'll just have to talk with the mechanic tomorrow — and you may just have to tap into the "rainy day" savings — that's why we've been putting a little money in there every month."

Dave was able to collect himself, and he went to bed grateful for his wife and his marriage.

Dave is generally a strong person, but: **Even the strongest of us sometimes get overwhelmed.**

Life sometimes sends its challenges to you in piles. As a matter of fact, Dave was also going through the stress of a move and the pressures of simultaneous deadlines of several projects at work. Fortunately for him, though, he was prepared. He had invested a lot of time and energy in his marriage (his second), and his wife was there to support him when he needed it. It wasn't the content of her advice that was most helpful, though it was a perspective he needed to hear. It's that she was there for him. Life was making a number of demands on him, and she was there to supply emotional support. It's like on the early versions of the VW Beetle, back in the late 1950s. They did not have a gas gauge on them, so when you ran out, you reached down and threw a switch to kick in the emergency tank. Dave's wife was his emergency tank, supplying fuel to his engine so he could perform better as a father, as a worker and as a human being.

Recall what I mentioned in Chapter 1 — that you can understand the idea of balance in terms of having a variety of tools available to you as you meet the diverse and unexpected challenges that will come your way. It's not just a matter of having money in a savings account to pay for a car repair, no more than it's being in good physical shape for when you have to run through the airport to make a connection. It's more like cross-training, where preparing for two events can help you with a third. Dave's family crisis over his son's divorce was helped by his wife's compassion. So was his financial stress over the car repair bill. He had other categories of his health that he could draw upon when he needed to do so. He had put gas in his emergency tank, just as he had enough money in his savings account.

Supply and Demand

It's helpful to think of situations when we "lose it" — some people prefer to call it "stress out" or "freak out," "melt down" or "go ballistic" — in terms of supply and demand. Stress (or overload, melt down, or whatever you call it) occurs when demand exceeds supply. In other words, when the situation demands something of you, be it energy, resourcefulness, skills, time requirements, creativity, patience, tact, courage, wisdom, money, support, or whatever, that exceeds the supply you have available. In order to solve this kind of problem — and one of the main points in this book is that it's a lot easier to prevent it than it is to fix it after it occurs — you may either decrease the demands or increase your supply. **Shorten the trip, or put more gas in your tank.**

Before I discuss a few ways you can do this, let me make another distinction. Some of the demands are external — imposed upon you from the outside. Your boss, for example, may be a total pain. Some of them, however, are internal. Your own sense of high standards may, at a certain point, be working against you because it throws your life out of balance. I'll give you a few examples of this later in the chapter.

It also helps to see your supply in terms of external and internal factors. You may go to external sources to meet a challenge, much as Dave turned to his wife or Greg, in Chapter 1, turned to a circle of friends. Or you may increase your supply of internal resources — such things as your physical health and vitality or your own psychological health. Chapters 4–10 of this book will discuss more fully how to increase these external and internal supplies.

Four Options

Here are four ways to prepare for life's inevitable stresses:

1. Reduce External Demand

This would seem to be the simplest choice. **Sometimes you just take on too many responsibilities.**

You over-promise or over-commit, and this puts you under a lot of pressure. You agree to attend a meeting at work when your attendance will not benefit you or the goals of the meeting. You plan a family trip where you have so many visits with relatives that you will spend all your time driving from one to another. You volunteer to chaperone a party at your kid's school, even though you have already committed yourself to help coach your son's soccer team, and you have a major presentation to make at work. You don't allow enough drive time to get from work to the restaurant where you are meeting your spouse because you promised your boss you would finish that report. You have a rare day off from family obligations when your spouse takes the kids to Grandma's for the day, but you promise to attack some household chore you hate instead of taking some well-deserved personal time.

> *A friend of mine who has the resources to stay at a hotel, spent two weeks at his elderly parents' condo in Florida with his two young children. He figured he would save money. At the start of his vacation his wife and one of his sons got sick. The "vacation" began with his 8 year old vomiting in the Detroit airport. He tried to catch the projectile vomit in his hands and then by accident ran into the ladies room to wash off. He spent the next week taking turns nursing different members of his family and asking his hard-of-hearing parents to turn down the volume of the TV. He called me after a week and said, "What was I thinking? I need a vacation."*

Reducing external demand is not always so easy. If you are stressing out because of the new assignment your boss added onto your workload, to tell him or her that you really don't think you can handle it right now is a little like career suicide. If your kids ask you to follow

23

through on your promise to take them to the zoo on Saturday morning, but you were planning to use the time to get caught up on some paperwork for the office, or perhaps go work out at the gym, then telling your kids that you are sorry, but you have other priorities is perhaps not the wisest choice either. As these examples suggest, it's not always so easy to say no to external demands. In some cases it makes very good sense to do so, but for high-performing people who want to be good parents and who want to succeed at their jobs, it's not always easy to pull it off.

How can you tell when reducing demand is the right thing to do? The answer sounds simple, and it is. Just say to yourself (or your spouse, or your colleagues at work, or even your boss), "Wait, let's think things through. What would be the most intelligent thing to do here, given all of the conflicting demands?" Ask yourself, **What is the best use of my time?** I am usually impressed when a colleague at work says something in a meeting to kill an upcoming unnecessary meeting that someone thought was necessary. Wasting our precious time with things that someone else thinks are important and urgent does not make a lot of sense. **As adults we have this marvelous ability to see into the future.** We don't get it right all the time, but we can be remarkably good at it. We are usually better at seeing into our kids' future than our own. "If you keep doing that with your model dinosaur, you're going to break it." "If you stay up all night, you are going to be tired the next day." "If you don't study, you won't do well on the test." It's pretty easy to do for other people, but not so

24

easy for ourselves. But we can and do if we stop for a second and think, "Wait, let's think things through."

> *Here's a personal example. My 10-year old son, Ethan, is an excellent tennis player. He really enjoys the game — except when he is losing. When that happens he gets very upset, sometimes bursting into tears on the court. You can imagine how this makes my wife and me feel when we are watching him. He plays in a number of local tournaments every year, but after one of his recent meltdowns, we got together and decided that he should not play in any more tournaments for a while. The mess caused by that kind of demand was just too much for everyone. It was becoming a total drain on our lives. I said to our friends, "We got together and decided," but the reality was that my wife and I decided and Ethan went along with our adult wisdom — which sometimes happens. He was confused and didn't know what he wanted to do, so we used our wisdom and experience to overcome his indecisiveness. We helped him to reduce external demand, and it is working out for all of us. The problem of his falling apart when he is losing is still there, but it's far less frequent and much more manageable.*

The result when you keep hurling yourselves into the whirlwind the result is what we psychologists call a mess. Jan and I – this time – saw the future, and we avoided the mess. A colleague of mine sees the problem this way: **A mess results when your obligation exceeds your commitment.**

In his language, (M = O > C). Most of us know the feeling. You agree to do something, so you are obligated to do it, but you don't really commit yourself to doing it. Chances are, one of two things results. Either the task remains undone but you feel this horrible, nagging drain on your energy ("I really should be cleaning the garage now because I told my wife I'd do it this weekend") that undermines your performance and enjoyment in whatever it is that you are doing. Or you go ahead and fulfill your obligation in a half-hearted way. I have a friend who regularly agrees to run errands, including shopping, with his wife, even though he may have pressing commitments related to his work as a writer. So while he is shopping with his wife, he would really rather be at his keyboard — which is where his mind is. She picks up on this fact without much difficulty, so she feels rushed and understandably annoyed. He feels obligated to accompany her, but he does not feel committed. He should have seen this coming.

The solution, and it's easier to say than to put into practice, is to get your obligations more in line with your commitments. **Obligate yourself to do things that you are committed to doing.**

When you say you are going to do something, then do it whole-heartedly, without thinking about the something else that you really should be doing.

This is where seeing the future comes in. Plan. Before you agree to take on an obligation, be sure you are committed. My wife and I do this fairly successfully — though like most so-called experts I manage to screw up pretty often. **Decide what's really important, and then figure out what course of action will most likely get you there.**

If what is really most important is to have a relaxing vacation, then don't make yourself have to rush to make airline connections. You may gain a few precious hours by taking an early morning flight, but if that means trying to rouse sleepy kids, getting them and yourselves packed and presentable, and then fighting your way through the inevitable rush hour traffic around the airport — then why not take the noon flight?

The most successful executives are excellent at screening out the unimportant stuff. In fact, they often have executive secretaries whose job it is to do a lot of that screening for them. Trivial or irrelevant phone calls are deflected. Junk emails are deleted. You might have encountered such a secretary on the phone – one who can be a real pain in the butt if you are the one being screened out, but great for screening out people wasting your time.

Few of us have an executive secretary working for us, so we have to do the same thing ourselves. **Activate the executive assistant in your brain.**

You know the drill from dealing with those dinner-time phone solicitations: Just say, "Not interested!" and hang up. It's sometimes harder to do this to other invitations to obligate yourself when you don't feel committed, but the principle is the same. It may mean deciding that your son does not need to sign up for both early morning hockey practice and Little League football. One activity per season should be plenty. It may mean opting out of that meeting where you have no constructive role to play, no value to add. And it may mean declining to attend your spouse's high school reunion when a little foresight says you will both have a better time if you are not there. Or — and this one can be touchy — declining to take part in a family gathering that you don't really have to attend.

Sometimes the answer is to delegate. Executive coaches tell business executives this, and it's no less true at home than it is at the office. Sure, some jobs you can't delegate, but some you can. Think about whatever it is that you hate to do, that you probably aren't very good at doing, and that you see as a waste of your precious time. Get someone else to do it. For me, one of the things that I really don't enjoy doing is mowing lawns. It was after mowing the lawn one precious Saturday morning that I decided that life is too short. I decided never to mow another lawn again. We bought a home with very little lawn, and I confess to getting a great deal of satisfaction when I work in my home office and look out the window at the neighborhood kid behind his lawn mower. For other people it may be home plumbing repairs, worthless meetings, business dinners, etc.

Of course, delegation often involves trade-offs, especially when family members are involved. "I'll deal with the garbage, you deal with the cooking." "I'll take the kids to soccer practice, you handle Cub Scouts." It helps if you have something valuable to bring to the trading post. The key is to work out a deal that works. **A deal that is bad for one party is bad for both.**

> *My wife Jan and I figured out a solution to mealtime and cleanup. It took us a while to figure out a division of responsibilities that works for both of us. During the week she takes care of most of the meals and the cleanup. On the weekends, however, Jan is not to lift a finger for cooking and cleanup. That's my share — breakfasts, lunches and dinners. Another couple I know has worked out the cleanup part by doing the dishes together, by hand – she washes, he dries – and for them it's a good bonding and talking time. Do whatever works for you and your family.*

Demands placed on you that you have no control over are, of course, a different story. There are plenty of times that we are told to do certain things that must be done immediately. There is no negotiation, no saying, "Not now." **But whenever there is an opportunity to**

get out of a burdensome demand that is truly unnecessary, take it.

It is interesting how things happen. As I was writing this, I got a call asking me if I would fly to Australia for 10 days to do some work. The clients were requesting me, and my schedule appeared open. It's an important piece of work, but it would make heavy demands on my time and energy. Quite frankly, I was very tempted to say yes. What I told them is that I wanted to think about it. Somewhere there is wisdom. I'd like to discover it. I postponed the trip until it was more convenient for me and my family.

Every case is different, of course, and as I said, you have to use discrimination in figuring out how and when it's appropriate to reduce external demand. But we are the species with the big brains, so our responsibility is to use them to pause and think things through.

2. Reduce Internal Demand

The demands that we experience are sometimes the result of internal pressures rather than external ones imposed by other people.

We can simply ask too much of ourselves, throwing our lives seriously out of balance. High internal standards are, of course, an important hallmark of high-performing people. It's an internal demand that leads you to paint that corner of your room just right, even though it is very unlikely that anyone will ever see it, or to make your bed every morning even though nobody knows but you.

Internal demand makes a writer fuss over the wording of a sentence just for the sake of doing it well, even when the time invested is way out of proportion to the impact on readers. It's high internal demand that has a high school biology teacher continue to read about research in molecular biology even though the results will have only a marginal impact on her teaching. She simply demands, of herself, that she keep up in her field. Or it's the grandparents who make the special effort to invite the grandkids over to connect with them. And it's high internal demand that draws successful business leaders to continue to read the latest books on leadership even though they are already at the top of their game. These demands to be the very best are what separate high-performing people from the pack.

No one gets better by luck. Think of Tiger Woods, who has enormous physical talent for golf but still runs and works out to keep himself in top condition. He is also, not coincidentally, the one who goes to the driving range after playing 18 holes in a tournament just so he can work on a problem in his swing. In fact, anyone who goes to the driving range has some internal drive to improve. All high performers have internal demands that drive them to improve.

Sometimes, however, these internal demands can go too far, throwing your life out of balance. **Life is not about perfection.** If your drive to make one or more aspects of your life perfect is creating the kind of pressure that leads to an imbalance, then re-evaluate your internal demands.

31

I know a golfer who was pretty good but did not enjoy playing. His problem was that he put so much internal pressure on himself to be good that it undermined both his performance and his enjoyment. His solution was to work briefly with golf psychologist Bob Rotella to reduce those internal demands, and now he is playing better than ever. More important, he is enjoying himself when he plays. **The point is to understand when it's OK to lighten up on yourself.**

When is it important to sustain those high internal demands, and when does it become destructive? The answer here, as it was when I discussed external demands, is to use our powers of discrimination. Say to yourself, "Wait, let's think this through." It's harder to do this with internal demands than it is with external ones. You can't say, "Not interested!" and hang up the phone on your own internal voice. But with some good self-coaching, you can do better than you are probably doing now. All that is required is a little dialogue with yourself using your most intelligent self. Ask yourself what is realistic, what is reasonable, what makes the most sense? If you find yourself using words like "always" or "never" or other exaggerated stupidities, chances are you're creating unnecessary demands. Very few things do we **have** to do. Just think about it.

3. Increase External Supply

The main point through most of this book is that we can all do a lot more to increase our supply — of energy, emotional strength, creativity, vitality, money, perspective, friendships, wisdom, options — in order to meet the challenges that we are bound to meet. Most of us have a hard time reducing demand. Our high internal demand has contributed to our success as high performers, and so we are reluctant to let go of that strength. And the high external demands are not likely to go away at our bidding. Your boss probably won't say, "OK — I'll come back with this new project assignment after you're through with your nap." **The other strategy is to increase supply.**

Let me give a quick preview of some ways to increase what I call our external supply.

- Nurture relationships with family members to whom you can turn for support.
- Connect with people who can help your career.
- Sustain friendships with positive, optimistic people.
- Locate and work with wise mentors.
- Save some money.

Again, more on these in later chapters. Suffice it to say that a number of people, stereotypically males, see themselves as the Lone Ranger. That role model may work to a certain extent, and self-reliance is indeed a noble virtue. But if what we are really interested in is high performance combined with feelings of satisfaction and balance, then our challenge is to increase our external supplies so we can turn to them when we need to. I am incredibly grateful that I am capable of going to people who know a lot more than I do for help.

A good example of a person who did this is champion bicyclist Lance Armstrong. Many people are aware of his story — how he overcame testicular cancer to go on and be a repeat winner of the 26-day Tour de France, the most grueling and prestigious bicycle race in the world. In his autobiography, *It's Not About the Bike*, you can see that he has always been a tough guy with a lot of internal resources — his discipline and his willingness to sacrifice for his goals to name just two — and he needed them all. What we also see is that he did not hesitate to reach out to external resources as well. When one well-respected doctor suggested a chemotherapy regimen that would mean he would never ride again, he tried other doctors until he came up with a course of action that worked for him. While doing this he cultivated a small network of close friends and supporters from the biking world and from his family, relying on them for emotional and psychological support. With the help of a nurse he was able to keep his attitude positive and constructive. He had some money saved as a resource, and he negotiated a supply of additional money as well as extended insurance coverage to keep him going. He was also in great physical condition (except, of course, for the cancer), and he drew upon this resource to get him through chemotherapy and to rebuild himself athletically. No, we can't all be Lance Armstrong, and we may not all be battling something as ruthless as cancer. But in our own way we are all like Lance because we have to draw on every possible resource to cope with life's challenges. **The more resources we have the better we handle adversity.**

Many years ago an executive named Ron found out his daughter was very ill. The doctors said she would die. There was no cure. He didn't accept the verdict. Using the same strategy as Lance, he relied on his friends for support, his job for distraction, his family for wisdom, his religion for faith, his mind for perspective and his exercise routine for relaxation. He had been a careful steward of his money so he could afford to fly her to places for experimental treatments. At this point, 15 years later, she is doing great. The doctors call it remission. It wasn't one thing that got him through, it was many.

4. Increase Internal Supply

Another good way to increase the supply of gas in our tank is through cultivating some of our internal resources. **One of the main advantages of choosing to increase your internal supply is that it's entirely within your control.** You don't have to depend on an understanding boss or spouse, and you don't have to spend energy connecting with family and friends. Instead, you work to build up your own strengths. This emphasis on self-reliance is also one of the main disadvantages of meeting challenges through increasing internal supply: There is nobody else to blame.

Most of this book explains how to increase your internal supply. This strategy is proactive rather than reactive. We generally will reduce external or internal demands only in response to some kind of overly stressful situation, but we can increase external and, especially, internal supplies in advance. And the great part about doing this is that you feel better, happier, more productive, and more successful in the process, whether or not you ever have to dip into those supplies in response to a challenge. I enjoy working out, whether I'm preparing for a marathon or not. I'm a happier person when I use positive self-talk, not just when I'm trying to convince myself not to be discouraged.

I mean several things by increasing internal supply.

- Take care of your physical health, the body in which everything else operates. (Chapter 4)
- Take care of your psychological health, by which I mean your attitude. (Chapter 5)
- Take care of your social health. This is "internal supply" in that you need to have the attitude of being a good friend, not just surrounding yourself with good friends. (Chapter 6)
- Take care of your spiritual health. Focusing on your highest ethical standards and living your core values can provide you with a tremendous resource. (Chapter 10)

Often the challenges life sends our way are a mix of internal and external, and so are the resources we need to deal with them.

J.C. is a friend who was an executive in the auto industry. He fell victim to an internal demand that was imposed by an outside policy. Several years ago the company implemented their "ABC Policy" where, by design, 10% of the executives were given the grade of A, 80% B, and 10% C. Those who were awarded Cs were given one year to improve their rating or they would be let go. This policy understandably created a lot of anxiety and fear, especially among people like J.C. — white males in their 50s. J.C. had to last two more years at his company before he would be vested with his retirement benefits and, given the company's commitment to affirmative action, he was afraid he would not make the cut. The kicker: People would be graded by colleagues often on their own work teams. It was like *Survivor* except you did not go home to appear on *Letterman* and *Good Morning America*.

To top it off, at about the same time, J.C. developed cancer. But he told me that the job stress from the ranking system was worse than the cancer. His father-in-law had lost his job several years before, and as a result his retirement benefits were lost along with his health insurance, and his savings drained. Fortunately for him, he was saved by a friend who was able to get a job for him. J.C. saw the parallels with his father-in-law, and he didn't like what he saw.

Fortunately for him, J.C. responded well to his situation, working hard to balance the seven areas of healthy living while at the same time getting successful treatment for his cancer. He has a great relationship with his wife, who supported him by reassuring him that things could be a lot worse and pointing out that his skills and experience would help him land another job, if it came to that. He also had a 22-year-old son in whom he could confide.

This kind of family support was important because J.C. could not confide in anyone at work — he was competing with them for grades and jobs. Fortunately, J.C. was a strong enough man to admit his fears and concerns, and to ask his family for this kind of external support.

J.C. was also saved by his great sense of humor. Never one to take himself too seriously, he was able to set his ego aside. His wry wit would crack everyone up, usually because he would say out loud what everyone else was thinking. People would complain about the ranking system and then J.C. would say, "Well at least I don't have cancer. Wait, I do have cancer. What a drag."

J.C. was also saved by the simple fact that he had disciplined saving habits, and he had set aside a safety net: enough money to live on for 6 months, in case of calamity. And he diversified his savings — another technique I will discuss later. This was an important part of what I am calling his external supplies.

Fortunately, the calamity never happened. The AARP filed a lawsuit that led to the end of the ABC Policy as discriminatory on the basis of age. I can't simply say here that he reduced his internal demands, for the ABC Policy created much of his problem just as the AARP resolved it. But J.C. also worked to get a grip on his fear and anxiety, seeing how he was generating it in response to his situation and then learning what he could do to take control of his response. By the way, after surgery and radiation there is no sign of the cancer one year later.

Secrets of the Obvious

- Reduce external demands when they interfere with what is really important to you.

- Have the guts and the intelligence to say "No"

- Challenge internal demands that add unnecessary pressure

- Cultivate your external resources — friends, colleagues, family members and money

- Cultivate your internal resources — your physical, psychological, social and spiritual health

Chapter 3

Progress, Not Perfection

Lucy is a perfectionist and proud of it. She graduated from college with a 3.9 grade point average, and that A- in Freshman Composition still rankles her. She went on to get her degree in medicine, and she is a standout in her profession.

Her success, however, has come at a cost. She achieved her academic success through lots of late-night studying. But she was far from a grind in college — she also enjoyed the dating and the parties that are a part of college life. Unlike most of her classmates, however, she would come home from the parties and put in a couple of hours with the books. And then in the morning she might go for a good run to clear her head and get those endorphins pumping. She drove herself, and it paid off with a great job at a major university health care system.

Lucy's drive continues now that she is the mother of two young kids. Deeply committed to her career, she also loves her children dearly and wants to be there for them the way her mother, a single parent who worked out of her home, was

41

*there for her and her brother. She knows
she needs to work full-time in order to do
her share to meet her family's financial
goals, so she gets up at 4:45 a.m. in order
to get to the clinic by 6:00 and put in two
hours on her paperwork before she starts
seeing patients. Her husband has agreed
to get the kids up and off to school and
daycare — and Lucy feels guilty about
that, though she knows it's only fair. With
luck, she can sneak in a run before
retrieving her daughter from daycare,
unless parent-teacher meetings or ballet
classes intervene.*

*By late afternoon she is usually exhausted.
She is very concerned about nutrition for
herself and her family, but often she is just
too tired to cook. She does it anyway,
though, or calls her husband to bring
home a take-out. Sometimes it's pizza, but
she feels guilty when this happens.*

*At night, when she and her husband have
checked over their son's homework and
both kids are finally in bed, she and her
husband collapse on the couch in front of
the tube. Housework will have to wait for
the weekend. Is there a soccer game on
Saturday? When is that ballet recital?
When will she get the laundry done? Will
she have time to go running and how is
her husband doing? And on a bad day this*

very high-performing woman asks, "Why do I stink at everything I attempt?"

Lighten Up!

It's not easy being perfect at everything — work, parenting, marriage, physical health, and emotional health. Lucy is doing great at most of them, but she is nagged by guilt because she falls short of her goals. She does not exercise as much as she should, does not eat as well as she should, does not earn as much money as she should, does not keep as clean a house as she should, and is not as available as a mom and a wife should be. And she does not look out for her psychological health as much as she should.

This is quite a burden of unhappiness for an extremely successful person.

Hey, Lucy — Lighten up! **Life is too short to be shoulding on yourself.** Let's face it! She's more together than 99.9% of us.

Of course, Lucy is not always like this. She is justifiably proud of her career successes, the charm and achievements of her kids and her husband. And she knows, in a non-arrogant way, that she radiates health and vitality. But all too often she gets caught up in the spiral of negative thinking that I just described. There is no reason for anyone, especially her, to put herself through that kind of misery, even for short periods of time. But we all do it, and all too often.

My very wise neighbor, who is a finance professor, explained to me an expression in probability theory called Stochastic Dominance. It states that the probability of success in any endeavor increases with effort. Now that is brilliant! Isn't it obvious that you'll be more successful if you work at something? The focus of this chapter is simple: **Do something to move yourself in the right direction, even though you may fall short of perfection, and then celebrate the something that you do.**

Talk is cheap, and negative talk can be very destructive. Recall again the seven areas of healthy living:

1. Physical
2. Psychological
3. Social
4. Work
5. Family
6. Financial
7. Spiritual

There is a tendency to think that unless you do all of them well, you're a bum. Not only is that not true, saying and thinking it is also counter-productive to being successful. And besides that, it makes you feel bad — and who needs that? Lucy needs to examine the way she perceives her goals and her relationship to her goals. Knowing Lucy, though, she would probably feel bad about how poorly she did at that task as well.

I once had a very bright and successful executive in a workshop say, only partly in jest, "Well, I'm lousy in 1, 3, and 5, and sorely lacking in 2 and 7. All I have is my job, number 4." He was exaggerating, of course, but he illustrates what I am talking about here. The whole point of this chapter — and your life, for that matter — is that it should be about **progress, not perfection.** That particular fellow was in fact kidding, but he admitted to being dissatisfied with his own level of progress in each of these seven areas. He is currently a CEO of a Fortune 500 company. When I visited him recently, he said, "I still remember those seven areas of healthy living. I'm not much better, but I'm still trying." He's being quite modest.

The Gap

The human mind has a tendency to focus on the gap between what we want to do and what we wind up actually doing. Let's say, for example, you want to lose 10 pounds. If you lose 1 pound, your mind could say, "I'm such a bum; I can't even lose 10 pounds." It would be much more positive and intelligent to say, "Good for me — I lost a pound!" If your goal is perfect weight or good health or great marriage or financial security — that's great. **You should celebrate any small step you take toward any of your goals.** Feel grateful, be thankful, and don't beat yourself up about how you fell short of your goals. And make certain you don't beat yourself up for how poorly you are not beating yourself up.

In the story that opens this chapter, Lucy is working very hard to achieve perfection at work and in her home — certainly worthy goals. And she also wants to stay in good physical shape — also very important. But the problem is that she is beating herself up because she is falling short of perfection.

A famous author, speaker and executive coach, Dan Sullivan, calls this "Living in the Gap." By this he means living in the space between the ideal that you envision and the actual goals you have accomplished. The problem with living in the gap is that we are forever feeling a sense of incompletion and thus are disappointed in ourselves. It's very subtle — though Lucy is an exaggerated example of the condition — and it pervades everything we do. **Nobody ever finishes everything they write down on their daily to-do lists.** There is always something more to do; and yet most of us focus on what we didn't accomplish on a given day rather than on what we did. I have a friend who adds things to his daily list after he does them, just so he has the satisfaction of crossing them out. Though he may seem to be foolishly obsessed with scorekeeping on his list, he does have a point. By focusing on the number of crossed-out items on his to-do list, he creates an appreciation for what he has actually done. He uses the list as a way to look ahead to his daily goals, but then also as a way to focus on real accomplishments.

If we understand the importance of these seven key areas of healthy living, we can appreciate that **any effort** — I repeat: **any effort** — that we give toward any of these should be considered time well spent. **Without effort there is no possibility of success.** Obviously, the challenge is to balance the demands of all seven in a way that works for each of us. Not perfection.

Lucy seems to be focusing her attention on the gap between the amazing things she has actually achieved and the impossible goals she has set for herself. In spite of all her accomplishments, she is not as happy as she really could be. Maybe somewhere in her life she has learned that "happy" means "content," and "content" means "lazy." So it's best not to allow yourself to be happy. That is just plain stupid. **What we're after is both success and fulfillment — however we define them.**

The Key to Misery

It's easy – insist on attaining perfect balance in all seven areas. Why is *that* the key to misery? Because attaining perfection is an impossibility.

> *I have a close friend who is a very good and very unsatisfied golfer. He is very serious about the game and very disappointed about how he plays. He continually focuses on his mistakes and lost opportunities. But he is a 3 handicap! He's really, really good! If you asked him on any given day, "How'd you play today?" he will never say, "I played great!" His standards are so high that his enjoyment of the game suffers enormously. There is no possible way that he can hit every shot perfectly — even Tiger loses a few tournaments a year. But my friend expects to score well every round. And he does score well, but his way of looking at his*

score and himself disappoints him. I don't think he would feel much better if he parred every hole. Somewhere in our life we have learned that it's good to set high goals, and we should feel bad when we fail to achieve them. This is the key to being miserable. My friend is also a good husband, a good father, and a good friend — a truly good person. But none of these things matters to him when he shoots a poor round — poor for him, I should say.

What is true for my golfing friend is true for each of us in all seven areas of healthy living. **There is no way we can be perfect performers in all areas.** Our goal should be to do the very best we can and enjoy ourselves enormously in the process. This may seem obvious, but it appears that very few of us have figured it out because it is so obvious. It's weird, but being slightly disappointed in ourselves seems quite appropriate to most of us. Maybe that sense of disappointment, like my friend's dissatisfaction with his golf game, is a way to say to yourself and to the world, "I'm really better than this." The problem is, of course, that we as human beings are notoriously poor judges of our own performance. We tend to be either too hard on ourselves or too easy.

The key to the seven areas of healthy living is not to add seven more things to your daily to-do list — which is seven more things you probably don't have time for in your already busy life. It's not seven more goals that make you feel bad because you fail to reach them. Instead, it's a framework for how you live your life. Are you working in a healthy way? Is your family life healthy? Do you keep a spiritual perspective? These are not add-ons to your life: They *are* your life.

If you look around and watch people you will notice that many of them are not having a good time. This is also true for many of us, but it's easier to see it in others, of course. Next time you stop at a coffee shop or at a restaurant, take a seat by the window so you can observe people on the street. You will see people scowling, looking irritated, and walking quickly. Many seem to be distracted or even irritated about something. Maybe it makes us feel more important to be that way — you know, that "I'm thinking about very important things" look. When you come across a person who seems incredibly relaxed, someone who obviously enjoys what he or she is doing at the moment, it feels very refreshing. This is the case because it feels good to be in the company of people like that but also because it's out of the norm. Doesn't it feel like they are in on a secret? They are.

The Secret

I suspect that one of the reasons that these people seem so happy is that they are not living in the gap. They are not focused on what they **didn't** accomplish that day. The perfectionists who are reading this chapter may be thinking, "Yeah, these are the lazy bums who never amount to anything because they don't have high enough standards." But I'm not saying that we shouldn't have standards. I'm not saying we shouldn't try to be better, or that we shouldn't raise the bar. In fact, I'm saying just the opposite.

Here's the key: If we continually raise the bar in terms of our performance goals in these seven areas of healthy living, and each time we do we try a little harder to get over that bar, this extra effort improves our performance, and it generally makes us feel better as we do better. But if we **don't** get over that bar, celebrate the bar we **did** get over.

If your goal is to live a more spiritual life, you should acknowledge and celebrate **any effort** on that behalf — a minute of meditation that you never before stopped to take or a conversation with a friend or colleague about what is ethically the right thing to do in a certain situation. Or even when you decide to place that quarter you found in front of the counter in the tip jar instead of in your pocket. You may not be living your life like a saint — in fact, you probably won't. **But your effort is its own reward.** The reward comes from the inherent benefits in whatever kind of healthy practice you have accomplished, plus your feeling of appreciation for doing better — for getting over that bar, however high or low it may be.

> *The other day I was playing golf with a man I'm just getting to know. Ten years ago he left the ministry to become a financial planner — an interesting career move, by the way. He has a healthy family life, three boys, a wife, a dog, and two homes. He took up golf two years ago, and*

he's intelligent enough to take lots of lessons. But what impressed me the most about playing golf with him was his attitude. He was so incredibly positive about his game. Every shot created a new opportunity for him. He must have reminded me 10 times that day to stop and appreciate the beauty of the course, the day, and how great it was to be doing what we were doing. He radiated gratitude. I, on the other hand, was mostly focused on the lousy score I was going to get because of that stupid triple bogey on that easy par 3. I know some of you are thinking, "I'd rather be the guy with the 3 handicap mentioned earlier." Maybe — but think about it.

Effort and Grace

What that important-sounding theory of Stochastic Dominance tells me is that we should at least make some effort to do something. Perfection is not the goal. As the title of this chapter suggests, if perfection is the goal then you are doomed to failure, and failure often means you stop trying. No, the point is to try, and to enjoy yourself in the process. In the next chapters of this book I will give you some idea about how you can do something in each of the seven areas of healthy living. **The probability of success in any endeavor increases with effort.** There are tons of things we can do or are already doing.

There is an ancient expression that describes how a spiritual seeker attains enlightenment: **The two wings that allow the bird of enlightenment to take flight are grace and self-effort.** And it's only through self-effort that one can woo grace. We can't rely on grace alone, or good fortune, luck, good genes, or whatever you want to call it, to get us through. It takes both. A friend of mine suggested I call this book "Effort and Grace." **Our job is to put in the Effort and Grace will come.** We do the basics of tilling the soil, planting the seeds, watering and fertilizing. The fruits of our labor are not within our control, but effort is.

This is true for all of the seven areas of healthy living. You do need luck or good genes or market conditions or the right breaks in your career. But self-effort in every one of the seven areas of healthy living can woo grace. Lance Armstrong wasn't "lucky" to win the Tour de France. He worked his tail off. Any success you have in your life isn't due to luck, either. You have been, are, and to some extent will be successful in all of the seven areas. Appreciate that success. And obviously, with more effort you will be more successful. **Do something.**

I find that it's helpful to look at your life or your day in terms of how your time is spent fulfilling the goals that you set or the dreams that you have. Remember, the goal is not to add seven more things to your daily to-do list. **The goal is to live your life with clear intention and purpose.** Yes, the workout time or the time spent in meditation might be seen as add-ons to your schedule, and so will time you decide to spend with your friends or your family. But think about it: Does it make sense to say, "I really don't have time for a great marriage at this point in my life"? Or, "It would be nice to be a more ethical person, but I'm just too busy at the moment. Maybe on my deathbed . . ."? Or how about, "My job really stinks, but I can't take the time to improve what I do at work"?

Try thinking about it this way: You are already engaged in all seven areas of healthy living, in one way or another. You have a relationship with your family — for better or for worse. You have an attitude and approach to your finances. You have a relationship with your body — even though it might be one that involves driving one block to get a Big Mac and fries. What I am suggesting is not that you add a new to-do to your life as much as it is to improve the quality of the to-dos that you are currently doing. These seven areas of your life are a great framework for setting goals. **The key is not to evaluate your life against these seven and give yourself daily performance reviews, but to use them as a framework for organizing your life.** They are reminders of what's important. As you walk through your day, as you're driving your car, as you're daydreaming in meetings, you can contemplate your life through the filter of these seven areas.

- Am I eating right today? Did I get enough sleep last night?
- That issue is really irritating me — what's funny about it?
- Do my buddies have the kind of positive energy I need, or do they drain my battery?

- What about my job isn't working, and is there a way I can delegate it?
- Have I spent some quality time with my family lately?
- How much have I put on my credit cards this week?
- I need to call the Red Cross and make an appointment to donate blood.
- Am I keeping my perspective?

These are not separate and distinct, obviously. Going for a walk with your spouse is as important for your mental health as it is for your family's health and your physical health. I know that there are some perfectionists who would say that now all you have to do while on that walk with your spouse is talk about the family budget, God, your career plans and have a couple of friends join you and you could knock off all seven at once.

Obviously, that's not the point. These are not items you can check off of your to-do list. Nor are they things you ever completely accomplish in your life. **The key is not to let any of them atrophy or wither from complete lack of attention and focus.** If you let them atrophy, it's just plain harder to get them back in shape. When you look at someone who has completely let himself or herself go, it's just going to take more effort for these people to get it together, but it's still possible. **Don't wait until you're a mess. Start now.**

My wife and I are friends with a couple who are very successful on lots of levels. Besides being quite nice people, both of them are physicians on the faculty of the medical school. They have two kids, a dog, and 17 sheep (they live in the country). It is their second marriage and they are both determined to do it right. Whether they apply these principles consciously or not, they have managed to balance the enormously complicated demands of their lives with tremendous coolness. We've been on trips with them and hung out with them, and quite frankly they live their lives well. They are not perfect. And they'd be the first to tell you that their lives are not in perfect balance. But they know that's not the goal. Their goal is to raise their kids, contribute to the world, treat their friends like family, and their family like friends. They're doing a great job. **It is not impossible; it just takes work.**

Secrets of the Obvious

- Avoid "Living in the Gap"

- Focus on your successes not your failures

- Perfection is never the goal

- Your effort will increase your chances of success

- Use the seven areas of healthy living as a framework for living your life

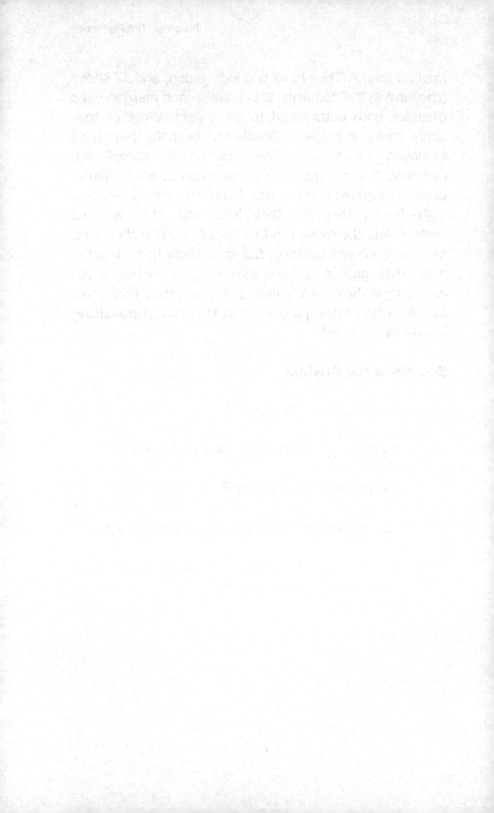

Chapter 4

Physical Health

Cindy looks up from the three law books sprawled open on her desk to glance at the clock on the wall of her office. Ten o'clock — her usual bedtime; but not tonight. She sighs and pours herself a cup of coffee. "I know I drink too much of this stuff lately," she says to herself, "but I need it to keep me going late at night."

She has been very busy researching a big medical malpractice case she will be litigating in a few short weeks, and she finds that the quiet of her office at night is her most productive work time. She has been able to make it home to fix dinner for her family — though sometimes she grabs a take-out or orders pizza. But then she turns over bedtime duties to her puzzled but obliging husband, usually saying, "I owe you, big time" as she heads out the door. She sips her coffee and chews on a breakfast bar, wondering just when and how she will repay him. Her partners at the law firm seem very pleased by her dedication.

Cindy is glad they are pleased, but she is a lot less glad about the disruption in her routine — with no end in sight. The trial may go on for months, and after that there will be more. It's the life of a young attorney trying to make a career. But there is a cost. She still gets up early in the morning, but she finds herself too groggy for the morning run that had been an important part of her life for years. Now she doesn't have time. The coffee keeps her going at night, and she often relies on a glass of wine to help her to sleep. But even though she is usually tired, she doesn't sleep all that well, and it's all she can do to drag herself to the coffee pot in the morning. Running is out of the question. She tries to take a run on the weekend, but she feels guilty about sticking her husband with the kids again after he's had to do all the nighttime duty with them.

She gulps down the rest of her coffee and places her mug decisively on the table. Back to work. This is important stuff: medical malpractice.

We are all athletes — you, me and Cindy in the story above. True, some of us are better athletes than others. Although I did complete the Boston Marathon a few years ago, at the finish line I was not surrounded by Olympic coaches seeking my services. And all of us are better at some athletic endeavors than we are at others. Some may specialize in jet-lag adjustment, others in entertaining a room full of squirmy middle-schoolers. There is no way my brother-in-law could handle the demands of his overseas work if he didn't take care of himself physically. We are all athletes because we depend on our physical bodies to do whatever we think is important to do, from running a race to litigating a law case to running a department meeting.

Because we are athletes, we need to take care of our bodies. Like it or not, it's your body that has to stay awake and alert during the business meeting or that gets you out of bed on a Saturday morning to take your son to his game. I know that when I get sick I'm a fairly useless human being — though I can fake being functional for a while. A Boston-area management consulting firm advises its new hires, "Get in shape!" as a prerequisite for the arduous travel schedule demanded in the competitive business world. If you only think of your body as the vehicle that carries you through the various tasks and adventures in your life, then it's important that you change your oil regularly, perform other routine maintenance, and keep some gas in your tank.

Get in shape now. A high-performance athlete doesn't just show up for the big game figuring he or she can get in shape as the game unfolds. Middle-aged weekend warriors may do that — these are the ones you see limping with pulled hamstrings or dislocated joints or, worse yet, being wheeled through emergency rooms following heart attacks. Professional athletes spend the off-season getting and staying in condition for the long season and, ideally, peaking for the big games. They know that if they are in shape they will perform better, and injuries are far less likely. Cindy, the hard-working attorney, may not realize that she is an athlete, too. And while it may be necessary to make some short-term sacrifices in terms of sleep, and the many other sources of nourishment in a healthy and balanced life, she needs to realize that her body needs to be prepared for the "big game" trial. And more seriously, she needs to realize that it's dangerous if her late-nights-with-coffee-and-skip-the-exercise routine becomes a way of life. She probably knows this, but like all of us, she needs reminding.

Looking after your physical health includes lots of simple things you can do as part of your regular maintenance so you are ready for the little surprises that life sends you: the sudden deadline at work, the illness in the family, the car accident, or the computer crash that destroyed your hard drive. Your physical health won't bring the contents of your hard drive back, but it will make you better able to deal with the situation. By the way, last month my hard drive was totally destroyed by a computer virus. Going for a run was an extremely helpful strategy for getting perspective on this minor inconvenience. No, I did not have my address book or files backed up. I do now. Like it or not, that brilliant mind of yours, that sensitive soul, is for the time being stuck in what Plato called the prison of the body. So you might as well take care of it.

Here's how. By the way, the points that follow aren't prioritized. They're just points:

Sleep

Get enough sleep. Not just once a week, but on a regular basis — every single night. How much? That depends on the individual. Most people need about 8 hours, but some need only 6 or 7. Some, and this probably includes a number of teen-agers, need a bit more. You can probably tell you are not getting enough by the way you feel when the alarm clock goes off in the morning. One researcher claims that the fact that you are being awakened by an alarm clock indicates that you are not getting enough sleep. I suspect that includes a lot of us.

I used to think I could get by on about 6 hours a night. But I learned that I'm much more functional with more sleep, and when I get 8 hours I feel really great. **Ever notice how crabby and groggy you are during the day when you don't get enough sleep?** That you are not your usual scintillating self? Even if you don't notice, other people probably do, and they may be kind enough to mention it to you.

> *I remember when my twin boys were first born. For the first few weeks they were home, my wife and I got very little sleep. Actually that is an understatement. We got almost no sleep. I remember being in such an altered state that the day and night blurred into each other. It was like we were in some kind of euphoric cocoon. We were so sleep deprived that we didn't know what was going on. I wasn't able to work very effectively, but it didn't really*

matter to me. The feeling of nodding off with one of those little blobs on my chest was something I will cherish forever. During the first few weeks of my sons' lives I would say that sleep was really quite overrated as a necessary bodily function. I was actually in quite a blissful state of mind. For a while. Eventually the lack of sleep caught up to me and I had to return to reality. Dozing off at work in the middle of a meeting is usually a bad sign. Everybody needs sleep.

How do you make sure that you get enough sleep? **Go to bed on time.** I'm a busy person — just like most people. This means I have to do some serious planning to get my eight hours. Go to bed on time. Don't eat a big dinner at 9:30 at night. Skip *Letterman*, or if you must, tape it so you can watch the show the next day. And when you get in bed — turn off the stupid TV. Really — if you miss one of those programs, what have you really missed? If you have coffee with your dinner, make it de-caf. This does not make you a wimp, nor does passing up that nightcap that may put you to sleep but may also wake you up at 3 in the morning.

If you are Doing Everything Right and still aren't getting enough sleep, then get some medical help. A good friend of mine has a sleep disorder called sleep apnea, which means he wakes up constantly throughout the night. For years he suffered from the condition until finally he dealt with it. A little common-sense planning, however, can help most sleep problems. Make it a priority. **The**

bottom line is to get enough sleep so that you feel rested and refreshed.

Sometimes, of course, you are going to have to cut short your sleep. Your child awakens in the middle of the night. Your boss springs a deadline on you, or you have to fly to Australia for a meeting. It's Final Exams, or whatever the equivalent is in your life. You have "crunch time" on the job with a pressing presentation to prepare. Or your house burns down. Whatever. When this happens, then you do what you have to do to deal with it. Most of us have probably pulled more than one all-nighter when in college in order to crank out a last-minute term paper. You do it, and you get through it. My point is that you can handle these crises if you have regularly been getting enough sleep, and when they have passed, you should go back to getting enough sleep. You'll feel better, and you'll do better.

Water

Drink a lot. A whole lot. More than you might think. That's 64 ounces of water per day. For readers who did not major in math, that's eight 8-ounce glasses. And don't cheat by trying to count your coffee and alcohol. Both of them are diuretics that actually remove more water from your body than they bring in. Drinking 12 Diet Cokes is OK, but it's probably better to drink 12 glasses of water. And caffeine does make you tinkle more.

Here's the deal with water: Most people don't drink enough. Even though nutritionists and performance coaches tell us that we need a minimum of 64 ounces of water, our bodies often need more than that and it is hard to tell. **We should be drinking water long before we're thirsty. If we're thirsty, it means that we're already dehydrated.**

Why drink so much? Because it's good for you. Most of you know the benefits of water, but in case you don't, here are a few: Water

- Carries nutrients
- Aids digestion and elimination
- Regulates body temperature
- Helps metabolize fat
- Improves skin
- Has no fat, sugar, caffeine – and it's free

High-performance athletes know they need to keep hydrated in order to enhance their performance. You should, too. You will feel more energized, increasing your capacity for doing whatever it is you want to do. No, it will not change your life. But it will help. When running a marathon, the single most important nutrient you must consume is water, tons of it. It will help you, too — whatever kind of marathon you are running in your life.

How do you know when you are not getting enough water? This one's a bit tougher than sleep, because you don't always feel thirsty from water-deprivation the way you feel groggy from sleep-deprivation. You can't simply say, "It's not hot and I'm not sweating," because we lose a lot of water through exhaling as well as through sweating, and we need almost as much on cold winter days as we do in the summer. And, coffee drinker or not, we lose it through urination. One simple test of whether you are drinking enough water is to examine your urine. If it's not clear in color, then you are probably not drinking enough. By examine, I mean look at.

But there's an easier test: Measure your consumption. No, you don't need to carry a measuring cup to the drinking fountain. But most bottled waters are sold in handy plastic containers (that probably cost more to produce than the water itself — but that's another story). All of them, conveniently, tell how many ounces of water they contain. So it's easy to keep track. Keep a bottle in the refrigerator at home or at your desk at work. I actually prefer mine at room temperature because it's easier for me to drink it that way. Whatever. Just drink the water. If the price of bottled water makes your jaw drop in astonishment, then buy one bottle and refill it from the tap or from your neighbor's filtration system.

If you are reluctant to be one of those people who conspicuously carry a water bottle to the movies or the mall, to the bathroom and the bedroom, then you can simply make it a point to drink at least a glass with every meal (that's in addition to whatever else you are drinking). The idea is to do what you can to move you to a more balanced and healthy — in this case I mean hydrated — life.

For those of you who don't like to drink water — do it anyway. **Go get a glass and drink it while you finish this chapter.** In fact, the next time you pick up this book, get a glass of water to go with it.

Balanced. No need to go nuts about this one. Don't say to yourself, "My God, I neglected my water the last five days! That means I need to drink 48 glasses today!" Just keep your water intake in mind, and if you're like most people, drink a bit more of it than you probably do now.

Smoking

If you smoke, you die. You already know this.

Just one little reminder I heard from my medical school professor friend: The Rule of Two. It takes two days for the nicotine to leave your system. It takes two months for the microscopic hairs (cilia) to be replenished in your lungs — their absence creates the smokers cough. It takes two years for your lungs to return to normal. None of these facts impact many smokers' decisions to stop. They have heard it all. But if they do decide to stop, it will make an enormous difference in the quality of their health.

Nutrition

How you eat, when you eat, what you eat and why you eat obviously impact your health and your performance.

First let's talk about *how you eat.* Have you ever noticed that when you wolf down your food you tend to eat a lot more? It takes a while for the food that you put in your mouth to reach your gut to tell your mind that you're full. So a simple thing to remember is to chew your food slowly and occasionally taste what you're eating. You'll probably eat less. Have you ever had the experience of eating so fast that you can't remember what you just ate? "Who ate all those chocolate chip cookies?" Slow it down.

When you eat matters. You probably already know that when you eat breakfast it speeds up your metabolism and prepares your body and mind for work. A good breakfast tells your body, "We are not in the fasting mode today, and more food will be coming, so it's OK to get moving." You may not know that eating late at night often disrupts your sleep and helps you get fat when those calories are not metabolized through activity.

Eating small meals throughout the day rather than the traditional three square meals allows your energy level to stay more constant rather than drop after the huge midday lunch or the grand slam breakfast. Try to go only a few hours before eating a small meal.

By "small meal" I don't mean a candy bar. Sugary snacks may give you a temporary lift, and I'm not saying that you can never have a candy bar. A small amount of chocolate, especially dark chocolate, may actually be good for you. But complex carbohydrates such as you find in an apple or a banana are much better for you.

What you eat not only determines whether you get and stay fat, but it also determines how you feel about yourself, how much energy you have, and to some degree how your brain functions. Food can make you sleepy if it's heavy or greasy and your body uses up a lot of energy to digest it with little left over to head up to your brain. Most of us know what we should be eating, but if we don't know we should make it our business to find out.

What you should be eating depends a lot on what your current condition is — if you are diabetic, or if you are elderly or a teen-ager, or trying to lose weight or build muscle mass, or pregnant or a nursing mother. It's important to change your diet if your condition changes, as many overweight ex-athletes can testify. But whatever your current condition, if you are trying to maintain a good healthy diet, you need to know what you're eating and what the effect is on your system.

Food is made of three simple things: carbohydrates, protein, and fat.

- There are two types of carbohydrates, simple and complex. Simple carbs are the sugars that burn quickly in your system. Don't make carbs your main source of fuel. They burn too quickly.

- You should make sure you're eating a portion of protein with every meal. It burns longer, like hardwood in a fire, as opposed to the kindling of simple carbs.

- As far as fat goes, be aware of it, but don't treat it like a poison. Obviously, deep-fried cheese balls are not the wisest choice you could make, but as I said, the occasional candy bar or hamburger won't kill you.

By the way, a portion is not the size of a loaf of bread. A portion is an amount of food equal to your clenched fist or the palm of your hand. My brother in law, who is also a very healthy physician, has a rule: **Never eat anything that is larger than your head.** Oh, and remember, eat a portion of protein with every meal.

Why you eat has more to do with the emotional place food has in our lives. We eat because we're nervous. We eat because we're bored. We eat because we don't want to feel some emotional pain. ("I'd rather feel full than fully feel.") We eat to avoid dealing with someone or some thing. We eat because it's a habit. We eat because everyone else is eating. We eat to be social. Sometimes we eat because we're actually hungry. It's impossible to completely become conscious of why you're eating, but it is possible to become slightly more aware of why you're shoving that donut in your face — at the same time you are saying, "I don't even like donuts."

So stop and think — when you shop, when you are looking over a menu, when you stand in front of the open refrigerator at night transfixed in the light like a deer in headlights. Read the labels occasionally so you are aware of what you are putting into your body.

Understanding why you eat is a big step toward managing how, when and what you eat. And managing

69

your nutrition is a big step toward improving your performance.

Watch out for fad diets or supplements that promise you a quick anything. Create a way of eating with a lot of variety, one you enjoy and can stick with. The key is not to create another nutty diet that you can't follow. **The goal is not to have a diet at all, but to have a lifelong way of eating.** You actually have one now. Is your way of eating a reasonable one? If it is, great. My mother-in-law has been eating well her whole life. She adapts her diet when information becomes available. She's just smart about what she eats. Her grandkids call her – affectionately – "low-fat grandma." It's no surprise she's in great shape.

The goal here is not about dropping a quick 15 pounds before beach season. It's about sustaining a healthy life over the long haul — the kind that can get you through those inevitable tough short hauls. Again — put nutrition on your physical health check-list, right alongside sleep and water. **Remind yourself that you can probably do better, without becoming a health nut.** If you know that your eating habits are lousy and you have no idea where to start, get some help from someone who knows what he or she is talking about. If your finances were a mess you'd get help, so why not do the same for your nutrition?

Caffeine

Don't drink too much. It makes you wired and irritable. It stresses you out. It raises your blood pressure. It may interfere with your sleep.

Let me confess right up front that I love Starbucks coffee. I'm a Starbucks nut. If I walk by one on the street, it is always tempting to get another cup. I'm not quite in recovery yet, but I know enough to monitor myself, to sense when I'm getting uptight and jittery. I'm probably never going to quit my coffee voluntarily but I can moderate my intake so I don't drink too much.

How much is too much?

> *A friend of mine with high blood pressure went to his doctor, who asked him if he drank a lot of coffee. My friend said, "It depends on what you mean by 'a lot.'"*
>
> *"How many cups a day do you drink?"*
>
> *"Twelve."*

How much is too much depends on the individual. For some people, one cup will make them twitchy and cranky all day. Others require two cups in the morning before they register a pulse. Twelve cups is probably too much.

Here's a little secret about caffeine — a secret that everybody knows: It's addictive. It's not crack cocaine, and it's not even nicotine, but it's still addictive. What

71

that means, among other things, is that after a while you may find yourself requiring more and more just to feel "normal." This is something you can check in your own behavior.

The good news is that it's not all that tough to quit because of the many substitutes available — decaffeinated coffees or herbal teas. And don't forget water. But I'm not saying everyone should quit. If you sense that you may be drinking too much coffee, then take it down a notch by making an occasional substitution.

Some people — like Cindy in the story that opened this chapter — get into a sleep-caffeine cycle. You are very pressed by some assignment and feel you need a caffeine buzz to make you productive working at night. It helps, so you awaken groggy and need a bit more to get you off the ground in the morning or to give you a late afternoon lift. This means you have trouble getting to sleep the next night, so you need a bit extra the next day. You end up like a wired zombie.

My point, again, is to experiment a bit to find out what works for you. Keep checking yourself — your sleep patterns, your irritability, your quantities. A friend of mine uses a very effective method for determining whether he has had too much caffeine. When his upper lip starts to bead up with sweat, then he knows it's over the line. Another friend, a surgeon, can't drink any because it creates little shakes in his hands. You decide what's right for you. Just be aware of it. When you sense something is wrong, something is out of balance, then pull it back into balance.

Alcohol

Sorry, but I have to talk about it. **There is nothing wrong with drinking alcohol as long as it's done in moderation.** It can be a great social lubricant and quite tasty to boot.

Drinking a little bit is no big deal — unless you are an alcoholic. In fact, every once in a while you see news items about how wine is good for you, or having a drink at night helps your blood pressure. If you find yourself clipping out those articles and attaching them to your liquor cabinet or refrigerator, then you may have a problem. If you tend to drink a lot, especially to handle stress, then you almost certainly have a problem.

If you are an alcoholic, it means that your body is unable to metabolize alcohol like most people, so you have to avoid it altogether. You can find out a lot more about alcoholism from Alcoholics Anonymous. I don't want to understate the seriousness of this disease, but occasional drinking in moderation seems OK to me for most people. But be careful. Remember the AA joke that goes back about 3000 years: Denial is not just a river in Egypt.

Exercise

This one is really important. Exercise helps you improve the quality of your life as well as the quality of your physical performance. You feel more successful when you are in good physical shape — I know I do. And you look better, too — though we all know how shallow and unimportant that is. I know I do.

You need to be exercising for the rest of your life. That means from now until you die, at which point the need to exercise declines dramatically, along with the stress you experience.

All of these seven areas of healthy living are lifelong pursuits, but exercise is one that is tempting to let go. "After all," you might think, "I passed my physical education classes in high school. I'm done. Now I work with my mind." Maybe you do, but the interaction of mind and body is profound. While much has been made lately about the ability of the mind to heal the body, the reverse is also true: A healthy body can improve mental functions. A simple example: Did you ever try to pursue a complex thought when you have a toothache? A less dramatic malfunction of the body — stemming from not getting enough sleep, water or exercise, for example — can lead to loss of energy, stamina or alertness.

How much exercise? How often? Of course, this varies greatly from one individual to the next. It might help to keep in mind the acronym FIT: Frequency, Intensity, and Time.

Frequency: Ideally, maybe three times a week — though four or five times would be better. But the idea here is that you can probably do better than you are doing now if you just remind yourself that it's important. If for you this means starting out by taking a walk a couple of times a week, then lace up those walking shoes and head out the door. **Do something that you could call exercise 3–5 times a week.**

Intensity: Vary it up and down — pushing at times, and then easing up. I occasionally run marathons, and I realize that I can't do all my training on flat ground if the course is going to include hills. If you do, your body will learn that there are no hills in this guy's life. If you see your exercise routine, like all these aspects of physical health, as a preparation for the stresses and challenges of daily life, then you'd better get ready for some of those hillish days that surely lie ahead. **When you are exercising, make sure you push yourself.**

Time: Each session should be about 30 minutes — though allow 40 to include warm-up and cool down. And you may feel better if you allow time for a shower. Truthfully — don't do it for fewer than 30 minutes, or the benefits drop sharply. But then again, there are no hard and fast rules. **If you are currently doing nothing, than doing anything is an improvement.**

The body is very crafty when it comes to working out. If you don't vary your routine, your body gets so used to doing the same thing that it tries to do it as efficiently as possible, with as little effort as possible. **To get the most out of your work out, remember to push yourself and do progressively more miles, weight, or speed.**

Exercise involves heightened, intentional stress. If you measure the body of a person who is exercising, you would conclude, "This person is under stress!" But it's good for the body, especially if you allow time for rest and recovery afterwards. Intense exercise, then rest and recovery. This is true for Olympic athletes and professional tennis players, and it's true for all of us. Think of the tennis players at Wimbledon who, between points, fiddle with the strings on their rackets, maybe towel off quickly, bounce the ball, or take a few deep breaths. They are resting and recovering for that next really intense point. Do this during your workout. If you are on the exercise bike, push those rpm's for a while, then ease off. Then push again. It's called "interval training," and that's what high-performance athletes do. Do it in your workout. **Do it in your life: difficulty, then recovery.** As I mentioned earlier, people who run long distances can't just train on flat ground. If they're in a race and find themselves confronted by a hill, they can't just say, "Hey! I'm a marathon runner!" If they haven't prepared for hills, they will pay dearly.

The physical benefits of exercise are obvious and well documented — even though most people find it convenient to ignore them:

- Fewer sick days
- More energy and stamina
- Better sleep
- Increased metabolism
- Decreased body fat
- Longer life

There are also benefits that are more than physical:

- Increased alertness
- Better mood
- Strengthened libido
- Better "quality of life" no matter how you define that term

The second group of benefits is perhaps less obvious than the first. They are mental and even spiritual benefits. I feel good — and not just physically — when part of me wants to quit 20 minutes into my planned 30-minute workout, but as I push on to the end. I get a kick out of meeting my goals. I get a kick out of using a bit more of my potential, overcoming the Lazy Boy lurking within me. These kinds of kicks — these "life lessons" — transfer to other areas of your life. All of us have the ability to reach down and find something extra. This is a matter of mental and spiritual strength, but it can find expression in something as simple as a physical workout.

The stance you want to cultivate is a "Bring it on!" attitude to whatever life has to offer. No, you don't want to bring down catastrophes on your head just to toughen you up a bit. As I said earlier in this book, life is going to continue bringing you stressful situations — tough challenges that will call upon all you have, and more. **The only time your life will be stress-free is when you are dead.**

> *Remember my friend Greg back at the beginning of Chapter 1? Prior to his heart "event" Greg was riding his bike about 50 miles a week, both for his physical and his mental health. His life with Linda, suffering*

from a mysterious illness, was very difficult to say the least. He used the bike riding as a means of relaxing and coping with the pressures of a sick loved one. What he didn't realize was that the riding was creating an alternative route for the blood to nourish his heart. The blocked artery was being bypassed by tiny collateral blood vessels. The doctor who put the stent in said that the biking might have been what saved his life.

What kinds of exercise? Let's keep it simple.

Do some aerobics — something that gets your heart beating a bit faster, your lungs working a bit harder. The goal is to get your heart rate up to about 80% of capacity, and you can buy a heart monitor to check this. But even without that device, just get the heart-and-lung machine working, but don't kill yourself in the process.

Do some work with weights. It's called resistance training. Your local gym has all sorts of equipment to give a thorough workout to all of your muscle groups, but for most people that is not necessary. An inexpensive set of free weights can be all you need, especially when combined with some push-ups and sit-ups. My 70-year-old father-in-law has been working out with free weights for the past year and has seen amazing results. He was already quite fit but he is even more so now.

"But I don't belong to a gym," I can hear some of you whining. "It's too expensive, and it would take too long to drive there and back. And I don't have room in my home for any of that fancy exercise equipment. And besides, who wants to get all sweaty? And what about my hair?" All this may be true. So do what you can within your present routine. My wife hates exercise and has always hated it, but she knows it's good for her so she does it regularly. She realized one day that she would never come to like it, but it has become something as simple as medicine that she has to take. She understands that exercise has to be part of her life. I think she represents the feeling that all of us have sometimes. The benefits are too real to ignore. Diabetics take insulin, we take exercise. Nike has it right: **Just do it!**

A few cautions here: Don't overdo it. Don't hurt yourself. Remember that I'm talking about balance — living a more balanced life. And you don't want to turn yourself into an exercise junkie whose pilgrimages to the gym start to crowd out work and family. If you find yourself doing arm curls with your infant daughter in the evening, you are probably taking this too far. Don't get all stressed out because you miss a few days of exercise because of a trip or an extremely busy schedule. Don't feel, because you missed a week, that you need to spend a couple of hours killing yourself on the exercise bike as some sort of penance.   **It's not about guilt — it's about balance.**

A friend of Jan's is in great shape. She runs almost every day. In fact, without her encouragement I don't think I could have finished the Boston Marathon. We ran together for the last twenty miles or so with Julie setting the pace. Unfortunately, as great as Julie is in keeping with her exercise regime, her challenge is knowing when to cut back. She recently injured her knee. The treatment is to stay off the running until it heals. Do you think she is heeding the wise counsel? She knows better, but just keeps chugging along. There is a bit of Julie in all of us.

Relaxation

Just chill. Relax physically — at the end of the day or in the middle of the day. Right after the stressful event as part of "winding down," or just before the stressful event as a way to get "centered" and focused. It's important.

Sad to say, some people don't know how to relax. It may be because of the caffeine issues described earlier in this chapter. But there are some simple techniques.

- Get into a comfortable position, seated but not slouched into the chair like a tossed sweatshirt.
- Breathe slowly and deeply. Take air into the lower part of your lungs, using your diaphragm.
- Repeat this 4 or 5 times.
- If you want to take the relaxation a step toward meditation: Focus your attention on your breathing, which conveniently takes it away from the day's problems.

Take time to relax and recharge your batteries several times during the day. A lot of people are so busy running from here to there that they can't take a minute or two to relax. You can take that minute or two. If you are like most busy people, this does not just "happen," so you have to plan for it, or at least, be prepared to take advantage of any few minutes that become available for relaxation.

Remember to breathe. Breathe deeply. Breathe consciously. Breathe frequently.

Health Checkups

In order to be balanced in the physical area, there is one more thing we need to do with a certain amount of guts: Go to a good doctor. I'm not talking about doctors who will prescribe pills for anything that ails you, but health professionals who look healthy, who give sound advice, and who admit when they don't know something. **Don't be afraid to get two or three opinions about whatever you want help with.** I know it's a pain, but some doctors are great and some aren't. Find someone you can trust, and do not be afraid to go to him or her with what has been bothering you for years.

The other day I was sitting out on the deck in the summer time with a good friend. He looked at one of my feet and playfully moved his chair a few feet away, and said that the toe fungus on my foot was gross, revolting and nauseating. He was having so much fun being grossed out by my foot that he kept coming up with new disgusting metaphors for my infected extremity. It dawned on me that I had become so used to it that I really didn't want to deal with the fact that he was right. It was disgusting and I should get it

81

treated. The reasons why I have ignored it will be covered in the next chapter, but the bottom line is this: I have had a minor health problem for years and have chosen to ignore it. If you don't know you have a problem, that's one thing, but if you know you have one and don't do squat, that's just plain stupid. Make an appointment with a doctor and talk about the stuff you're too embarrassed to talk about.

Cindy's problem at the beginning of the chapter is not a simple one. Her career is important to her, as ours are to many of us, and sometimes this requires putting in some long hours. That means, of course, those hours have to be subtracted from something else in your life — your sleep schedule, time with your family, and your exercise routine are the likely targets. For short stretches of time you may need to shift your life out of balance in order to accomplish short-term goals.

My advice for her, and for people like her, is two-fold:

Minimize those sacrifices, for some of those things you are giving up — sleep and exercise, to name just two — are the very things that will enhance your attaining your goals. Cindy will be in better shape to win her case if she is a strong and rested athlete.

Seek balance in your overall life. If you are healthy — physically and in the other ways I discuss in the next few chapters — then you will be in better shape to deal with those stressful times that tend to knock your life off-center. Cindy will need to find a way to resume her previously healthy lifestyle after the pressures of the medical malpractice trial. She needs to attend to her own malpractice.

Secrets of the Obvious

- Plan so that you get enough sleep

- Drink plenty of water — at least 64 ounces per day. Watch caffeine and alcohol consumption

- Eat small meals throughout the day, with more fruits and vegetables and fewer fats and sugars

- Eat protein with every meal

- Exercise at least 3 times per week, 30 minutes a session, mixing weights and aerobics for the rest of your life

- Get regular health checkups, especially when you have a problem

Chapter 5

Psychological Health

There is a woman I know, Lenore, who is extremely bright, a great mother and wife, and a nationally recognized research chemist. I mention how bright she is because it's not her intelligence that is her challenge. She is a caricature of a pessimist. I'm certain she is unaware of how she comes across. I have never had a conversation with her where she doesn't complain about something — the weather, her clothes, how a teacher deals with her kids, how her kids behave. It may be something small or something large, but it's always something. In fact, when I see Lenore, it usually takes fewer than 5 minutes before she says something negative. The only thing excluded from her complaining is her work. Even when things are going well for her, she'll say something like, "I can't believe how well this is working — I'm sure it won't last. Every silver lining has a cloud inside, you wait and see." She's not nasty or mean. She's just absolutely convinced that the glass is half empty. For Lenore, like all of us, the world is as we see it.

A well-known story about an old Vermont farmer has a neighbor asking him if he's going to take some courses over at the agricultural college. "Nope," he replies, "I already know more than I can do."

There has been an enormous amount written in the last few years about how to attain good psychological health, and most of it is entirely true. Go to a garage sale or a used book sale at the library and you will see lots of those books being discarded. Why? The mind is such a complex thing that anything we know about its workings must invariably be complex. But at the same time, in our busy lives — lives that for most people are working out fairly well, thank you very much — it is difficult to implement complex changes in thinking and behavior. Lenore has spent a lifetime honing the skills of pessimism. So have we, in our own way.

For that reason I think it important to deal here with obvious stuff — things you probably already know, and things, with just a bit of effort, you can find a way to do. As you will see as you continue reading, there are no arcane theories here, no going back to your toilet training, no radical new theories about the nature of human thought, and no fancy diagrams showing how the mind really works. I'm not talking about the psychology of men in contrast with the psychology of women, or people at mid-life versus people who are young and on the make. Remember — these are secrets of the obvious.

Before I get to those secrets, let me mention a technique we need to use — one we already use now and then.

Pay Attention

A lot of us spend a lot of our so-called waking hours in a daze. We may be paying good attention to the boss speaking at the meeting, to the ball game on television, to what our spouse is saying, or to the group of squirmy teen-agers we are teaching or coaching. But we are not necessarily paying attention to ourselves and how we are thinking as we are doing any of these things. The fancy word for this is "metacognition," but I prefer to call it "paying attention." **It's thinking about what we are thinking about.**

It's not always easy to do. Being aware of other people's mental processes is not that uncommon — we do it all the time with our friends and family members, with folks we see on television or in the movies — but it's hard to apply the same awareness to ourselves. It involves stepping back to watch ourselves respond — to observe ourselves being stupid or defensive, generous or forgiving, angry or egotistical, or whatever we sometimes bring to the party. Usually this kind of paying attention happens shortly afterward, when we say, "What an idiot I was," or "I handled that crisis with good self-control." Sometimes when Jan or I are particularly levelheaded when dealing with one of our kids, I'll mention that we deserve a Ph.D. in childrearing for that moment. That's in contrast to the same parents acting like total fools the next moment.

Kids, by the way, are really good at saying out loud exactly what they are feeling. They haven't learned yet to censor what goes on in their minds. We, on the other hand, think this stuff so we don't say it out loud.

One technique we can use to help us stay tuned in to how our minds are working involves listening to our self-talk. You know what I mean by self-talk, either because you have read about it or you are used to listening to that little voice inside your head. It's pretty much always going on inside us, saying things like

- "Why does this always happen to me?"
- "Here comes the part where I always screw up."
- "She's doing that because she doesn't really like me."
- "I'm in a groove now, where all the good things happen."
- "God, this is fun!"
- "OK, so the next step for me is to . . ."
- "This is boring."
- "I hate this/him/it."

As I said, this kind of talk is going on all the time. The secret is to start to listen to it with a critical ear. **What kind of self-talk are we generating?** Can we produce a kind of self-talk that makes us perform better and makes us feel better? Obviously, we can and do already. It requires being a great parent, coach, friend, mentor, or wise sage — **to ourselves.** When you listen to anyone giving another person wise counsel, that's the model we need to follow. **The goal is to be wise — verbally, to yourself.**

With some effort we can focus our self-talk in a few distinct areas.

Being Stupid

Sometimes we do stupid things. We know they are going to be stupid before we do them, but we manage to turn our sensible self-talk volume way down low, and then we blunder right ahead. Sometimes people who behave this way are called "headstrong," though I find the term spectacularly inappropriate. Who's kidding whom? **Stupid is as stupid does.**

> *I recently went skiing with my family out in Colorado. We awoke one morning to nine inches of fresh powder — it was incredibly beautiful. Some of the young kids who were with us, veteran skiers in their late teens and early twenties, said, "Let's take a powder run through the trees — it'll be awesome!" I remember saying to myself, "Yeah, cool — I've always wanted to do that!"*

> *Now I'm a decent enough intermediate skier, but I know I can't ski in fresh powder, especially when it's a steep run through the trees. But somehow, caught up in the enthusiasm of these young people, my own reluctance to be middle-aged, or whatever, I managed to turn off the inner voice that was telling me, "Don't be stupid." So I found myself at the top of*

the run, scared to death, with everyone else flying off in a very big hurry. I had absolutely no business being there! I remember a cocky 18 year old giving me a tip as he sped away: "Don't look at a tree — you'll hit it." Thanks! I appreciate your advice.

Fortunately for what was left of my ego, there was one person — a 22-year-old woman — who was as incompetent as I was. She pretty much buried herself under the snow and inched her way down, and together we crawled through the trees. After about 45 minutes of this nonsense we used the walkie-talkie to summon help. (Bringing that equipment was one of the few non-stupid things I did that morning.) Eventually we made it to the bottom — embarrassed, sore and, mostly relieved.

There are a number of lessons in this story — lessons about ego and self-created stress. But the point I want to make now is about not listening to the "Don't be stupid" voice. I emerged from my little adventure on the slopes with a few bruises on my butt and my self-esteem, but sometimes the consequences of stupidity can be more serious. Think of the decision to drive two more hours at night on that family trip, even though you have put in 10 hours behind the wheel and your caffeine jag has your hands shaking. Or the decision to have a drink after work with that attractive person in the office, even though both of you are happily married. Or driving to work in a snowstorm when you have no business being out in such weather. Or having just a few drinks with the gang and then driving home. Or shoveling snow off the roof when the roof is icy. In all of these examples there is probably a voice inside shouting, "Hey! That's really stupid!" But you turn down the volume and go ahead.

Before I had kids I watched a friend with her two small kids. She bought them cherry-filled, glazed donuts, which they proceeded to spread all over themselves, each other, the car, and her. This was 15 years ago, but I remember vividly her words as she tried to clean up the mess. "What the hell was I thinking? I ought to have my head examined." I was amazed by the fact that she obviously knew better — but did it anyway. She could have examined her own head and paid attention to that inner voice. For whatever reason, she didn't that time. I don't think it's important to do therapy to discover why we don't listen to our own best counsel. There are a million reasons. **The obvious point is that we do manage to listen some of the time — we just need to do it a little more.**

Sometimes we are fortunate enough to have someone else say aloud what our inner voice is whispering. The other day I was playing golf with a friend on his course for the first time. He suggested that I not use a driver on a particular hole since I didn't need the distance and the consequence of not being straight would be costly. What do you think I did? Of course. I used my driver, belted the ball out of bounds, and had to listen to him smirk, "I told you so." I knew all along that I didn't need to use my driver, but something — maybe it was pride this time

91

— made me too stupid to listen to my own voice and my friend's. The fact that he said I was just like his wife didn't help, either.

Some people are blessed with a spouse who externalizes that voice, but this fact does not always make it any easier for us to listen. When an adult hears a cautioning voice, unfortunately the response is often one of defiance: "Don't tell me what to do!" Sometimes it's easier to reject someone else's voice out of a sense of personal independence than it is to reject our own inner voice. You know how it goes: "No man (or woman) is going to tell me what to do," or "You never let me have any fun." Suddenly the issue has shifted from your upcoming stupidity to the nature of your relationship. And there you are, defiantly juggling chain saws, telling off the auditor from Internal Revenue, or signing up your kids for ice hockey when practice is Saturday mornings at 6 a.m. sharp. It's much simpler to leave your spouse out of the stupidity discussion. **Our job is to practice listening to our own, or anyone else's, wise counsel. Period.**

Of course, there's nothing wrong with giving your kids the occasional jelly donut or challenging yourself with a difficult ski slope or golf shot. All I'm saying is that we can anticipate the consequences of a lot of these choices, so why not just avoid the messes we are not prepared to clean up? In other words, don't be stupid.

> *I was watching an ESPN program about a workshop for all NFL rookies. It was intended to help them cope with the*

demands of being in the NFL and the transition from college kid to multimillionaire professional athlete. The theme that went through every topic they covered was choices, decisions and consequences. It was a mantra they kept repeating over and over. Unfortunately, few of the players could remember the three words even one month later. The lesson could have easily been titled "Don't Be Stupid." They covered the basic truth of how every one of us is confronted with choices, which involve making decisions which will have consequences. Loaning money to friends, having sex with women they don't know, hanging out with unsavory characters, using drugs, etc., were all covered by the presenters. The fact that this was for NFL rookies was interesting, but the same principles apply to all of us.

We need to see the consequences of our decisions as much as possible from the sum total of our life experiences and other people's life experiences. The little voice inside our head that says, "maybe this isn't such a good idea" comes from a lifetime of making mistakes and learning from them. Even if we don't have the experience of doing something stupid, we can certainly know from other people's experience that it is stupid, and so we can choose to not do it. I've never taken heroin, but I know that it is not a good idea. You might be thinking, "Well, that's so obvious." Exactly! Think of the entire continuum of silly to foolish to less than prudent to stupid to unbelievably stupid things we've done in our lives. **To err is human; to not learn from the error is stupid.** Or as Cicero said, "Any man can make mistakes, but only an idiot persists in his error."

A friend has a five-year-old grandson, Lucas, who says grace before the evening meal. Part of what Lucas says every day is, "Help us to make good choices." He was obviously coached by his parents about what to say, but at some level he is learning about choices, and he is learning about listening to his inner voice, whatever its source.

In Perspective

Here's a letter that a first year student at the University of Michigan wrote home to her parents:

Dear Mom and Dad,

I love going to the U of M. I hope all is well with you. We had a little fire here last Tuesday, but I escaped through the bedroom window. The fire took everything, but the doctor says that the baby is going to be all right and I should be able to go back home in a few weeks.

My boyfriend Bill has kindly offered to let me stay at his motorcycle club with his friends until all the bandages are off.

Love to all,
Carol

*P.S. There was no fire. I'm in perfect
health. I'm not pregnant, and I don't even
have a boyfriend. I got a "D" in Chemistry,
and I just wanted you to take it in the
right perspective.*

The point behind this story should be obvious enough.
Are you really getting all bent out of shape because you
are having trouble getting the weather stripping on the
storm door? Are you stressing out because you can't
afford a new dock for that second home you have up on
the lake? Is your Sunday paper an hour late? Is that
miracle of modern communication, the Internet, a little
slow this morning? Do you find when you fly from New
York to Los Angeles in a matter of hours that you are
really upset by the quality of food that they serve on the
flight?

I don't want to sound naïve here. Some really terrible
things happen to people: cancer, automobile accidents,
rape, real financial disasters that disrupt family life,
chronic pain or depression. But getting a zit on prom
night probably does not qualify, nor does a "D" on an
exam.

**Our goal is to keep our perspective, which means
being able to distinguish the really important stuff
from the obviously small stuff.** Richard Carlson's
aptly named *Don't Sweat the Small Stuff* makes this point
clearly in the title. Use the "pay attention" technique to
think about how you are thinking.

In order to cultivate the attitude of perspective, it sometimes helps to look at others who have no perspective. It's certainly easy to see with kids. This morning both of my kids were crying real tears about something on the video game they were playing. It had to do with winning and losing and not playing fair and breaking promises and annoying each other and blah blah blah. How important was it in the scheme of things? Obviously, to them it was very important. They weren't old enough to know any better. Most of us adults are old enough to know better, but we freak out over things that we can't control or don't amount to a hill of beans in this world.

In the last years of her life, my mom was so much more mellow than she used to be. It may have been that she was approaching the end of her life. Or maybe she was always this wise and I never recognized it. I think it's both. Anyway, my mom had this great capacity to see the big picture. **What difference does it make that things didn't go according to the best-laid plans?** They rarely do.

I remember one time when I was sixteen. I came home totally freaked out that I had been in a car accident and wrecked the family Ford. The main thing my Dad was concerned with was that I was all right. He had the wise perspective.

My Dad showed the same wise perspective about 10 years ago when I was audited by the IRS. I was so freaked out. The kids had just been born, I had no experience with anything like this, and my accountant was not what you would call reassuring. I was imagining the worst. I remember Dad's counseling me in such a matter of fact way, saying everyone gets audited once in his or her life. It's a pain in the butt, but it's no big deal. The worst that can happen is you wind up paying them some money. It turned out well, and his wisdom and perspective were more than reassuring. They were good parenting, good leadership, good friendship, and good therapy. These are all about helping people get perspective. When we're in the heat of the moment, of course, we don't see the larger picture, but that's where wisdom comes in.

Obviously, keeping things in perspective is easier said than done, but here's the truth: We already do it all day long. **There are enough things in our life every day to get angry about constantly and we choose to overlook most of them.** Here's my wise counsel: Overlook a few more. As a colleague reminded me recently, **"It's just stuff."**

Your Sense of Humor

The advice to "keep your sense of humor" is much easier to give to another person than to take ourselves. Why?

The 19th century American wit Ambrose Bierce defined happiness as "an agreeable sensation derived from the contemplation of the misery of another," and he makes a good point. It's a lot easier to laugh at stuff happening to someone else. A lot of good news/bad news jokes are derived from this fact, jokes along the lines of: "A doctor says to his patient: I have some good news and some bad news. The bad news is that you have a terminal disease. The good news? I don't."

There is a second reason that is related to this one. It is very difficult to step back from ourselves, see ourselves as going through some really funny stuff — funny because we seem to be taking it so seriously but we are blind to that fact. I have a friend who is a very successful teacher but fairly inept when it comes to routine home maintenance. There is no big sin in that ineptness, except that he gets really angry when he tries to attach extensions to his downspouts without bringing down the whole system, or when he struggles to reattach a wheel that has fallen off his lawnmower. His wife sees how comical it is when he gets so angry, and she tries – with admirable sympathy, but not a lot of success – to help him see the humor. My friend can laugh at himself a week later, after he has calmed down, and he even enjoys telling of his amusing mishaps to his friends. He, like all of us, tends to forget to see himself as a humorously fallible human being.

The notion of applying effort to develop our sense of humor may itself seem quite ridiculous. "What are you doing, Harry?" "Oh, I'm working on my sense of humor." It's not the same as what we do when we work at something like the timing of our joke delivery or the wording of some witty remarks we're going to use in a speech. But a sense of humor does require a certain playfulness that can be cultivated. We all have the ability to laugh at the imperfections going on all around us — including our own mishaps. All we have to do is open our eyes. And don't take ourselves so seriously!

I enjoy people who have a great sense of humor, when they don't take themselves or the world too seriously. This is not to say that everything is a joke — quite the contrary. My wife and I were watching Colin Powell give a news conference six days after the destruction of the World Trade Center. He handled every question with honesty, directness and clarity. At one point a reporter interrupted him and he interrupted her back, saying in an exaggerated slow way, "Wait... let me finish...." But he did it playfully, which made everyone laugh. Then he said, "Now see what you made me do! I can't remember what I was going to say. What was your question?" Again everyone laughed. Then he answered every question with the same directness as before. Colin Powell was just being himself. Teasing the reporter, but also poking fun at himself amidst one of the most difficult times in all of our lives.

The point is to keep our sense of humor about ourselves no matter what happens. Pay attention to our own voice when we are taking ourselves so seriously by saying, "I'm not merely human with human fallibilities. I'm not going to fall in the dirt from time to time. And it's not funny!" Or " I'm very important" or "I'm very cool" or "I'm very smart." Or "I'm incredibly organized."

> *One time when I was in grad school I was on my way to teach a psychology class. While riding my bike down the street, a friend waved and I turned to wave back. I rode directly into three feet of freshly poured wet cement that was being*

99

fashioned into a large planter for trees. The cement was up to my thighs. The front wheel was completely submerged. Everyone was gathered around laughing except for the guys pouring the cement. They pulled me out, hosed me down, shook their heads at my idiocy, and recommended that I watch where I was going. What helpful advice. My friend just stood there smiling in disbelief. Soaking wet, covered in cement residue, I went to teach my class. The good news was that I was such a mess that it made for a hilarious class.

It really does help to turn the camera on ourselves. How would we look if we watched ourselves from the outside — getting so irate on the golf course or tennis court, or blowing the circuit breakers when we try to hang a ceiling light, or getting peed on by our baby boy when we try to change his diaper.

Here's a story that makes the point about humor in a different way:

Feeling Stressed?
Picture yourself near a stream...
Birds are chirping in the crisp cool mountain air...
Nothing can bother you here...
No one knows this secret place...
You are in total seclusion from the rest of the world...

*The soothing sounds of a gentle waterfall
fill the air with a cascade of serenity...
The water is clear...
You can easily make out the face of the
person whose head you're holding under
the water...
There now... Feeling better?*

People find this funny because of the nasty little surprise at the end. The story acknowledges our sometimes less than noble emotions, and it airs them out in the safe venue of a joke. If someone were to tell jokes like this all the time, you'd better call for building security. But in moderation it's just a way to blow off some steam and have a little fun by stepping back to pay attention to your feelings. **Always keep in mind that our sense of humor is a muscle, and it needs to be exercised at least once a day.** Even if it's just a quiet little chuckle at your own idiocy or someone else's. Just make sure you don't become a jerk in the process. Do yourself a favor: **Lighten up!**

Putting Yourself Down

We all know how toxic the negative self-talk can be; both the kind where you say what a loser you are, and the kind where you assume what a loser everyone else thinks you must be. Either one can be deadly. Think back to the skiing advice I was given right before I was going to take that powder run through the trees: "Don't look at a tree — you'll hit it." If you look at yourself as a loser, you will become one.

The message here: Time to get out of junior high, where everyone seemed more popular than you, nobody really liked you, and, besides, you looked really weird. In all probability only one of these was true.

I like to identify this kind of negative self-talk in terms of what Martin Seligman calls "The Three P's of Pessimism": **Pervasiveness, Personalization,** and **Permanence.**

While I was writing this book, I sent a proposal and several chapters to an agent to see how she liked it. There were three possibilities: She could say "Great! Let's send it out to publishers." She could say it's a bad idea and not worth writing. Or she could say that the idea needs some more work before it's ready to send out. I waited for a month for her to get back to me about my book.

If I were a pessimist — and I admit that I had some pessimistic thoughts during that month — I would have followed the three P's like this:

- **Pervasiveness.** It's not just that she doesn't like the book. That is obvious. The real problem is that nobody is going to like it and the whole idea is stupid. Her opinion represents the opinion of most agents and publishers. She's no idiot; if she thought the idea had any merit, she would have said so. This whole project was a dumb idea. What was I thinking?

- **Personalization.** The problem here is with me. It's not that she is busy with other people's books, or is taking her time to write some thoughtful and helpful suggestions for me. No, I sent her something so lousy that she doesn't know how to respond. It's me. I thought I had something of value to offer people, but really my ego just wanted to write a book that has been written 50 times already. I guess this just shows the truth: I just don't have what it takes to write a book.

- **Permanence.** This book is always going to be rejected. If I try sending it to other agents they will no doubt reject it, too. And if I publish it, it's doubtful that anyone will buy it either, because if she didn't like it, no one will. So I might as well not try writing another book ever again, because the same thing will always happen. Her rejection is the kiss of death.

It would not occur to a pessimist that she might just be on vacation, or busy with other book projects, or coming up with helpful suggestions. The pessimist might also conveniently forget that there is another agent who expressed interest in the book and is waiting to see the proposal and sample chapters. The fact is that she *did* get back to me and sent me a contract. Seligman spends his entire book, *Learned Optimism*, writing about this issue of optimism and pessimism. Here's an excerpt:

> *The optimists and the pessimists: I have been studying them for twenty-five years.* **The defining characteristics of pessimists are that they tend to**

> *believe that bad events will last a long time, will undermine everything they do, and are their own fault.* The optimists, who are confronted with the same hard knocks of this world, think about misfortune in the opposite way. They tend to believe that defeat is just a temporary setback, that its causes are confined to this one case. The optimists believe defeat is not their fault: Circumstances, bad luck, or other people brought it about. Such people are unfazed by defeat. Confronted by a bad situation, they perceive it as a challenge and try harder.

Again, the idea here is to pay attention to your self-talk. **If you hear the voice of pessimism whispering in your ear, identify it for the toxic force that it is.** As an exercise, try hearing what an optimistic voice would say. You may want to call in an optimistic friend or family member at this point, but even better, try calling up the optimist inside you. If you have to fake that voice at first, that's OK, but listen to what it has to say. Doing so will show you that there are always alternative ways to see your experience, and you have the power to choose which one you will use. Look at the exact same situation with the glass half full.

The son of a friend of mine was going through a divorce. He was only in his early 20s, and it was the day to move his stuff into his apartment. As he trudged through this painful transition, he commented on the way his life seems to never work out. And come to think of it, whenever he orders a pizza, they never have the toppings he wants. Even Kentucky Fried Chicken was out of chicken once when he went there. Clearly the universe was conspiring against him, and it showed in his posture and walk as he carried his speakers to the car.

He was seeing the world through the lens of his failed marriage, and he was personalizing what happened to him, as if the folks at KFC quickly threw away their chicken when they saw him coming. I'm not saying that there is any quick fix for him, "Hey, cheer up and get over it!" What I'm saying is that he can step back and listen to his inner voice, which at the time was probably sounding a lot like the voice of Eeyore in *Winnie the Pooh*. You know: "Don't worry about me — you guys go on without me. I'll just sit here in the dark waiting for someone to call. Life sucks and then you die." **Paying attention to that voice is a necessary first step to changing it. And we can change it.**

> *We just had dinner with some friends we haven't seen in a long time. The man shared that he hadn't been able to exercise for a year because he had his hip replaced. This guy used to run almost every day and play golf several times a week. When I asked him how he was doing with it he said that it's been hard but he's OK. He sees the world with the glass half full. "It could be worse," he said. "I could be dead."*

105

Take Charge of Your Emotions

A long time ago, the Roman stoic philosopher, Epictetus, born a slave, said, "If anyone is unhappy, it's his own fault." What he meant by these very unsympathetic sounding words has a simple truth to it. While we can't control all the externals that happen to us, we can, to a certain extent, control the way we respond to those externals. It takes a lot of self-discipline and self-awareness, but we can do it. Epictetus himself showed this self-discipline when he was being tortured by some thugs employed by the Emperor, Nero. As they were twisting his leg he calmly stated, "If you keep doing that, you will break it." And then, "I told you so."

Epictetus is a hard example for most of us to live up to, but we recognize the truth in what he says about controlling our emotional responses to the world. As he said, **"Man is not disturbed by things, but by the opinion of those things."** Of course it's hard to control our emotions, or our opinion of things in every situation, but there are times when you can make it work.

> The other day I was driving down the freeway late for an appointment, and as I was getting onto the exit ramp I pulled in front of a guy in a pickup truck. I could see him in my rearview mirror cursing me and giving me the finger. He pulled up next to me and continued to spew his vituperative rage at me while we waited for the light to change. I rolled down the window and listened for about 5 seconds as he cursed

me out with his veins bulging from his neck. As I drove off I wondered how long he is going to hold on to that fury. Will it impact his entire day? Will he let it roll off him like a bead of water on a duck's behind? I doubt it.

I'm making the assumption from the look of him that he has no idea that I didn't cause his rage. Granted, I clearly was wrong to cut in front of him. But what separates us from animals and children or less evolved humans is our ability to control ourselves. We don't poop in our pants and we don't have temper tantrums when things don't go our way – most of us, anyway.

The ability to control our emotions is both inherited and learned. There is actually a name for it: Emotional Intelligence. Daniel Goleman has written several excellent books on the subject. The main point of his first book is that the ability of people to understand our own emotions, empathize with the emotions of others, and control our emotions is a learned skill, and one that must be cultivated our entire lives. A related point is that the more emotionally intelligent we are, the more successful we will be in work and life. He has an interesting way of describing what happens when we lose our temper. The part of our brain that controls emotions is called the amygdala. When we lose it and can't seem to regain our composure, the amygdala has been hijacked. Eventually we calm down, but only after we've made a fool of ourselves. This is very different from the controlled use of anger to make a point.

> *One evening about 20 years ago, I was walking with my wife down a street in Ann Arbor. A man who was obviously drunk walked by us and insulted my wife. My wife said something appropriate to him like "Buzz off!" and he said "Bitch." The next thing I know, I, wise psychologist and stress management expert, am rolling on the ground with this guy yelling, "Apologize to my wife! Apologize to my wife, you jerk!" I've got the guy in a headlock with my arm across his mouth. I couldn't hear what he was saying — if he was saying something. This whole scene is happening in seconds. Luckily we let go of each other and said a few choice words as we went our separate ways. My wife couldn't believe what had just happened, nor could I. The last time I was in a fight was in eighth grade. Luckily, the only thing that was bruised was my ego.*

It's not that we shouldn't feel upset or lose our cool sometimes. But rather, we can do what we already do in tempering our emotional reactions of rage and anger — but do it more often and better than we already do. Currently, my kids are the perfect challenge for me to practice this. I don't lose my temper very often. But my kids can push my buttons so easily it's embarrassing. The good news is that I know it's about progress not perfection, and I don't expect myself not to be an idiot with my kids sometimes. I also know that with effort I can keep it together so much more now than even two years ago. A few days ago my son was freaking out on the soccer field. As he continued to cry and make a scene, a friend and parent of another kid on the team remarked at how cool I seemed to be as the coach tried to deal with him. I replied that he happened to see me on a good day, demonstrating a little bit of wisdom. Two years ago I would have been out of control, grabbing him, lecturing him, and yelling at him in an effort to get him to control himself. The out-of-control parent lecturing the out-of-control kid about the importance of controlling oneself: excellent parenting strategies employed by the expert!

Positive Self-Talk

Taking charge of our emotions also means taking charge of our self-talk and how we see the world. Throughout this chapter I have been saying that we need to listen to our self-talk because we are often a great source of wisdom and common sense — if we would only listen. But there is more that we can do.

If you catch yourself putting yourself down by saying things like, "I'll probably screw this up," or "That happened because I'm such a loser," then you can start to change your attitude by changing your language. When you start to say, "I can do this well," or "Things will be fine," your mind will start to believe what your words are telling it, and this can change the way you feel about yourself and about the world around you. And when you change the way you feel about yourself, the way you behave will change as well. Just in case any of you didn't know, how we see the world is a reflection of our inner state of mind. If we're in a great mood, people seem quite pleasant, but if we're in a foul, cantankerous and disgusted mood, people are jerks. **The good news, of course, is that with some effort we can change our own inner state.**

I remember watching an interview with a figure skater right before her free-skating routine. She said something like, "I'm confident that I won't fall doing that jump." This sounds like good positive self-talk, but it isn't. She is focusing on the act of falling. It's like "Don't look at a tree — you'll hit it." She fell doing the jump, of course. What sounded like positive self-talk was based on an image of failure. In the same way, if you say, "I'm not going to screw this up," the key language says, "going to screw this up," and that's what you picture. Instead, say something like, "I'm going to do this with grace and skill," and picture yourself doing it. Even though you may have some internal doubts, you can talk yourself out of those doubts. When you talk to anyone who has fought back from an illness, overcome a challenge, or dealt with adversity of any kind, the common thread that links every person's story is that they see the future as positive and successful. They picture themselves nailing the triple lutz. They literally see the future as they would like it to be. When they fall on their behinds during the practice jump, they know that falling is part of the process. But they see themselves winning, beating the disease, getting the job — even when there are setbacks in the process. There is plenty of research that shows that the most successful salespeople are not the ones who get few rejections. They are the ones who get the most rejections but have resilience and perseverance in the face of failure. **Hank Aaron still holds the record for the most strikeouts and most home runs.**

Obviously, I'm not saying that just picturing it in your mind and saying that you will make your goal happen will guarantee the result. Look at the alternative. Since we're talking to ourselves all the time, pay attention to what we are saying. We can and do choose what to say. We can choose to walk around saying, "Life stinks, and then we die." Or "Today I will experience gratitude for everything I have been given." Or "I'm going to be successful this time." Or "We can win this thing." Or...

There are many names for what happens when we lose our perspective, forget our sense of humor, put ourselves down, etc. It's been called "stinkin' thinkin'," "catastrophizing," or even "optical rectitus." The bottom line is that we can proactively cultivate the mindset of seeing the glass as half full. **The world is as you see it.**

111

Secrets of the Obvious

- Pay attention to what's in your head

- Don't be stupid

- Keep your perspective

- Cultivate your sense of humor

- Don't put yourself down

- Take charge of your own inner state

Chapter 6

Social Health

I've known Bob for over 20 years, and I cherish our friendship. Bob and I established a club that through the years we have allowed others to join. Greg and Doug are members now. We call it the Testosterone Movie Club.

Almost every Friday night we go out to a movie, one that our wives would not really appreciate. We root for the good guys, delight in the creative ways the bad guys are wiped out, and of course appreciate the love scenes for their artistic sensibilities. We shun any movie that is "well-crafted." We have so much fun with each other that even terrible movies are a blast because of our relationship. Sometimes we call a "red alert," which means that we can't have any excuses for not going out because two first-run action flicks have just been released. If one of us bails out with some lame excuse, like needing to spend time with our family, then he is put on "double secret probation" for however long we can milk the whole stupid charade.

Usually before the movie we'll review the week and talk about what's going on in our lives. What's so special for us is that there is no judgment, no pretense, no competition (except ping pong), and always lots of laughter. We can talk about our work without trying to impress. We can talk about our kids and wives without their having a clue. We can talk playfully about money and how one of us is making so much he should give the rest of us some. We can talk about our spiritual aspirations without sounding silly. We can talk about pain, uncertainty, doubt, fear, sports, politics, and that huge zit on one of our faces. Most of all, we can talk about anything we want.

People have written about the importance of friendship for centuries, yet in our busy lives it sometimes takes a back seat to the all-important work and family. Friendship feels to some of us like a nice thing but not that necessary in the grand scheme of life. Well, here's my big revelation about the obvious: **Friendship matters.** Just like all of the other resources in our lives, the ability to cultivate, nurture and sustain relationships beyond our immediate family members matters. A lot. As I get older and, I hope a little wiser, I've begun to appreciate the value of friendships that we have maintained over decades.

When you watch kids play, what is so amazing is that they are doing a million things that just wouldn't be as fun unless they were doing them with other kids. While I love to play golf, I just don't enjoy playing golf by myself. By the same token I don't love to play golf with strangers. There are only a certain few people I like to play golf with. For me it's more than golf. **It's fellowship.**

The same joy that kids have playing with each other is something that we as grownups long for. Since we aren't allowed to run through the woods throwing sticks and climbing trees, we have to find more sophisticated and cool games which have the same effect on us emotionally. I could never understand why a good friend of my Dad's would show up on Sunday morning to hang out and eat bagels and drink coffee. The neat part was the fact that he never called or asked permission to come over or made a big deal about it — he would just show up. Now I know how important that relationship was to both of them.

I remember a lot of valuable things that my father told me when I was growing up — and when I was an adult, for that matter. Here's one of his gems: ***"The most important thing in life is to be good with people."*** Being good with people can mean several things. At a cynical level it means manipulating people — the way a slick salesperson can get you to buy something you don't really want, or a smooth politician can manipulate you to vote a certain way. Being good with people can also mean being comfortable with people, being at ease and affable in any social setting. This is a bit less shallow than the first meaning, but it still doesn't get at what my Dad meant.

I see the heart of the phrase as having two meanings: **Be a good person to others, and be with people who are good for you.**

Good Company

There is an ancient spiritual teaching that advises the seeker to be good company and surround oneself with good company. What this means very simply is that if you're on a path heading to a goal then it makes sense to surround yourself with people who will support your efforts and not make your journey more difficult than it is already. This applies to all of us in our lives. We have lots of goals in our complex lives. We need all the help we can get in reaching those goals. If one of your goals is to live a healthy life, then hanging around people whose habits make it very difficult for you to do that is kind of stupid. On the other hand, hanging around people who will support you is smart. It's obvious that kids of all ages are influenced by the company they keep. It's true for us grown-ups as well.

> Last year my neighbor, Mark, and a friend and I decided it would be cool to climb Mt. Rainier. A friend at work described it as an emotionally, physically and spiritually enriching experience for anyone. We trained together during the summer, walking steps with 50-pound packs, and then we flew out to Seattle.
>
> The process is simple. You train with experienced guides for a day to prepare

you for the trek and to weed out those whose physical condition would put the climbing party at risk. The next day a group of 20 climbers and 5 guides hikes to a base camp at 5,000 feet. At midnight, in groups of 4 climbers to a guide, roped together, you attempt to climb the remaining 9,000 feet by dawn, then descend all the way back down.

The experience was everything my friend had told me, and more. Twelve people finally made it to the summit, but not before several climbers volunteered to turn back or were told to do so by the guides. At 12,000 feet the guide leading our group insisted that one of the men in our group was slowing us down and was jeopardizing the safety of the team. He dug a small ledge in the snow, pulled a sleeping bag from his pack and told the man to get inside and not move until we returned to pick him up on the way down. I was thinking, "I'm next." My fear was mixed with dread and hope.

To make a long story short, all three of us made it. But there is no way we would have if we hadn't been supporting each other the entire way. At every opportunity as we were slogging up the mountain we would ask each other, "How you doin', Mark?" "How you feelin', Harry?" "You OK,

Peter?" And every time one of us would lie back, "I'm feelin' great!" or, "I'm with you." As we were walking down, the guide confirmed what all of us felt. You don't climb a mountain without people supporting you. But, for me what was as great as the experience of summiting was the camaraderie of the journey. I told Mark that I truly appreciated his company. His sense of humor, his sense of perspective, and his sense of gratitude made the trip even more special. The guides asked us all why we wanted to climb, and Mark said, "Because I can. I see a lot of people who cannot." He's an orthopedic surgeon who works with spinal cord injuries. Mark is good company.

One of the easiest ways that friends can support one another is by expressing sincere appreciation. Say thank you. Each and every one of us likes to feel appreciated, and sometimes we don't feel that way unless someone tells us we are. It doesn't have to be a tearful, look-them-in-the-eyes, heart-throbbing experience — the kind with lots of background music. It can be light and funny. A colleague I work with has become quite a good friend. Both of us tease each other that when one of us does something nice, the other owes him a Hallmark card. We will never send one of those things; it's not our style. What we have learned to do is say, "Thanks, man." "You're welcome." It is another one of those obvious truths, but I know people don't express their appreciation enough. At least, I know, I don't.

Toxic People

Surrounding yourself with good company is as important as the food you eat or the thoughts you cultivate in your mind. Maybe even more so. Have you ever noticed that certain people are not good company for you or your family? If you were really trying hard to lose weight, it would not be very smart to hang out at the donut shop where people are stuffing themselves. If you want to keep your marriage healthy, it's not wise to hang out with people who put your spouse down. The quickest way for someone with a drug problem to get back into trouble is spend time with the old gang. What's that old expression, **"Lie with dogs, get up with fleas"?**

If one of your goals is to cultivate the kind of positive attitude that I talked about in Chapter 5, where you see the glass as half full and focus on your accomplishments, then it's pretty stupid to hang out with people who are sarcastic, mean, selfish and cynical, and who take great pleasure in criticizing, condemning and complaining.

I have a friend who teaches at a local high school. When he was promoted into a leadership position of department chairperson, he found he had to reevaluate where he ate lunch. The table in the teachers' cafeteria where he always sat featured a group of very witty and clever colleagues who were skilled at ridiculing the principal, the school board, members of other departments and students. The conversations were always funny and enjoyable in a way, but my friend realized that with his leadership goals of improving the climate of his department, he could not be sucked into that attitude. So he started eating elsewhere, with more positive people.

Your good friends are, in a way, your support group — just like AA, but maybe without so much smoking. They give you the wise counsel that any good parent, mentor, coach or shrink should give you.

Having a long history together is sometimes not a good enough reason to hang out with a person. What we really want in our friends is shared values.

I am not being paranoid in saying that there are some people who are jealous of you. They don't like you for whatever reason, and they can be quite nasty. They can put you down behind your back or just send you bad vibes. They either intentionally or unintentionally undermine you in subtle or not so subtle ways. They can take credit for your work, or even just outright steal your ideas. Your job is to smell this garbage and avoid these people like the plague. If you confront them, it will only create denial and more garbage. Hundreds of times in therapy sessions when clients would tell me about how certain people were treating them, I would remind them of an ancient saying I heard which I found helpful: There are 4 kinds of people in this world: those who are happy, those who are sad, those who are virtuous, and those who are wicked.

Toward the happy we should be glad for their happiness. Toward the sad we should feel compassion. Toward the virtuous we should feel delight. Toward the wicked we should be indifferent.

Just walk away. Don't try to convert them, change them, teach them, or scold them. You are not their parent, nor their shrink. Reasoning with an evil, wicked nut case is not going to work.

If you do decide to take them on because their crime or transgression or behavior is sufficiently disgusting, just make sure you have the right support. The right support can mean many things — including the authorities. The point is, don't do it alone. Even cops call for backup. Also, be clear about your intention. If you are just trying to extract a pound of flesh, it is probably a dumb idea. On the other hand, if you want them to know that you know what their game is, go for it. Be careful, though. There is an old quote about two people fighting in the mud. Both will come out filthy.

Obviously, every situation is incredibly complex. But when you sense that someone is treating you with real disrespect, unless you're a paranoid nut, you're probably right. This does not mean you should walk around being victimized by everyone who looks at you cross-eyed or take everything so personally. It does mean that you should listen to your gut if people are dissing you. There are lots of reasons for that. Some people are having a bad day, or are incredibly stressed, or just didn't notice you. **Some people are mean; avoid them.**

Jerks

Without getting into a deep discussion of exactly what a jerk is, I think we can agree that jerks are toxic, and we don't want to be one. We all know this because we don't like to be around them. There is something in their unabashed selfishness and arrogance that just turns us off.

Before you agree too quickly with this secret of the obvious, we might note that the jerks are not always "them." Sometimes the best of us can act that way. But let's just keep referring to these narcissists as "them."

We all know what they are like:

- They are sealed into thoughts about themselves, like a person in an imaginary bubble. Occasionally they stick their heads up to note with surprise, "Oh, look! There's somebody else out there!" But then they are back in the bubble, talking and thinking only about themselves.

- When they are taking part in a conversation and the other person is talking, their minds are busy formulating what they are going to say next rather than listening to what the other guy is saying.

- They are constantly thinking, "How can I make this conversation about me?" If you are telling such a person about the fatal illness of your mother and maybe seeking some emotional support from your friends, you suddenly find that the conversation has switched to an illness that she suffered from ten years ago, and look how brave she was and how splendidly she recovered. Once I saw a generic get-well card that captured this idea. It read, **"I had what you have — but worse."**

- They are like the person in the joke about the self-centered movie star who has been babbling about himself for a while. But he catches himself and says, "But that's enough about me — let's talk about you. What do *you* think of me?"

Some people are jerks; avoid them. And avoid being one.

Listening

The primary talent to cultivate to make you good company is a simple one: listening. By that I mean deep and attentive listening. **Look at people when they are talking.** Pay attention to what they are saying and what they are trying to say beneath their words. Shut up. Listen sympathetically, trying to see their world view if only for a while. You can always disagree or argue later on. When I was a full-time practicing therapist, many of the people I saw felt like friends to me. In fact, many of our sessions were conducted over lunch in restaurants.

Some of my former clients have become friends. I know some of you are thinking, "How desperate. This guy used his practice to troll for friends, how pitiful." It really wasn't that weird. Mostly what I did as a therapist was listen. Giving wise counsel or challenging some dumb behavior could only work if I were really listening. **People really appreciate being listened to.** It's so basic that it seems almost unnecessary to say it, but good friendship works that way. You appreciate advice from a friend who has really listened to you.

> *My friend Doug just called. He's in the midst of preparing for a difficult trial that starts in a few days. I heard the anxiety in his voice. He shared some of his fears and what a drag it has been to be waking up every morning at 5 a.m. out of anxiety. After chatting for a while and consoling him about the trial, he asked me what was going on in my life. I playfully shared that I was waking up at 4:45 a.m. from my anxiety about my own stuff. Then he asked what was really going on. I told him about a complicated decision at work, which actually involved an important legal opinion. He listened well enough to offer his wise advice, which turned out to be exactly the thing I needed to hear. He told me to go talk to a lawyer.*

A Third Place

Sociologist Ray Oldenburg argues in *The Great Good Place* that people need what he calls "a third place." The first two are obvious enough: home and work. These are, properly and necessarily, the central focal points for the time and energy of most people, although some — traditionally it's been women — have combined these two into the profession of "homemaker."

But these two, home and work, are not always enough, and Oldenburg says that everyone needs a third place where he or she can meet and socialize outside of the demands of work and family. Think of the neighborhood pubs in Great Britain, or the bar in the television program *Cheers*. The function of Starbucks is much more than drinking coffee.

It doesn't have to *be a place* — a restaurant or bar, a club or a coffee shop — but friendship does need to *have a place* in your life. It can be a group of people from work who do things together that have nothing to do with work. It can be a book group or a quilting group. It can be something like our Testosterone Movie Club. The point is to be together, and when the time comes when someone needs to talk, friends are ready to listen and support.

What I'm saying about the importance of friendships doesn't have to involve a group. It can just be some friends that you feel it's important to get together with every once in a while, maybe one at a time. And if you find yourself saying that you really value friendships but are just too busy to work them into your schedule right now, then you are letting your life get a bit out of balance.

Integrity

Say what you mean, mean what you say, and don't say it meanly.

Most Important Words

I want to return to the words of my father that I mentioned at the beginning of this chapter: "The most important thing in life is to be good with people." I don't know where I found this list of the most important words. I find it useful to keep the list in mind as a way to cultivate friendships. The words are no less valuable for family relationships, but I want to put special emphasis here on the often-neglected role of friendships in keeping our lives in balance.

The 6 Most Important Words: "I admit that I was wrong." These words are important for an obvious reason — humility. It feels great to be right all the time, doesn't it? Our pride or self-righteousness can be a real threat to relationships, for the obvious reason that if we are the one who is right, then the other person is the one who is wrong, and who enjoys being with someone who makes us feel that way? **We all make mistakes. So admit it when we do.** That makes us feel better and everyone around us feel better, too. Remember, though, to be sincere in your admission that you were wrong.

Don't just say it as a way to end an uncomfortable argument or to defuse an awkward but necessary confrontation. Most of us have pretty good built-in BS detectors, and we can tell when the admission is not truly felt. I guess this means that the first step is to actually recognize and acknowledge to ourselves when we are wrong. And then take the next step and tell the other person.

> *A friend and I have fun with this one. Neither one of us likes to admit when we are wrong. In fact, we'll go to great lengths to find ways of being right. We'll wait for just the right moment to remind the other of how we were right about something stupid. "See I was right, you should have used a nine iron." "The right lane is definitely faster than the left lane."*

The 5 Most Important Words: "You did a great job." These simple words are so important because we all like to feel that we are appreciated. It's a basic human need. We don't hear or say these words often enough at work because many bosses feel that the words might imply some lowering of standards. But we need to say them because people are so prone to focus on any negative criticism that is spoken or implied. We need to say them at home because again, who likes to be taken for granted? It could be a small thing — a minor home repair, a well-cooked meal — or perhaps a celebration of an achievement by a spouse or child outside of the home. The words show that you are considering and appreciating another person's life. Words like these can really cement a bond of friendship by lifting the relationship out of the realm of competition that dominates so much of life. You are also climbing outside of that narcissistic shell to acknowledge that someone else, other than you, is doing great stuff. Some psychologists have recently questioned saying words like these because they tend to establish a demeaning sense of hierarchy, with the boss dispensing praise down to the underling. But I think that *that* criticism is nonsense. **Just say it when you see it.**

The 4 Most Important Words: "What do you think?" These words, like the ones above, are important because they take you outside of your ego. They indicate that we actually care about what our friend (or family member, or colleague) is thinking. Through these words, we are taken out of the argumentative frame of mind that can lock us into defending our own point of view. The words suggest openness and curiosity about our fellow human beings — very appealing in friends. They are a demonstration of true respect. The next time you are in a meeting, watch what happens when someone is asked what he or she thinks. Their whole demeanor changes. "You mean you really value my opinion?"

The 3 Most Important Words: "I love you." This one might be difficult to say in the context of friendships, especially in America. The words bring up all sorts of romantic connotations that just don't fit well in friendships. But I think that true friendship has strong elements of love in it — not romantic love and not family love, but love just the same.

128

The question, then, is how to say it. It's difficult to say to a person of the opposite gender without sounding like you are making a pass. And it's hard to say it to someone of your own gender without sounding like you are gay — and making a pass. In marriages and families my advice is simple: Just say it. In the case of friendships, my advice is similar: Just say it — if it won't make either of you too uncomfortable, and if there are no misunderstandings. Or maybe, if the words are frightening, find another way to say it. No, not with flowers! Say it in a semi-joking way, like my friend and the Hallmark card. Or say it through your listening, your being there for your friend, your being good company. **Express it.**

My point here, in part, is that we can be open to this kind of depth in our friendships. We can say it, first, to ourselves, acknowledging how much we value the friendship. Once we are aware of this feeling, the expression may take care of itself. But if it doesn't take care of itself, find a way to say it.

> *Dick, an old college friend of mine, currently lives in Connecticut and works in Manhattan. On his drive home on Friday nights he will often call me from his car to chat about our lives. If he lived here in Michigan, he would make an excellent Testosterone Club member. Dick is a rare man who epitomizes the great qualities of a friend. He is a great listener. He has a great sense of humor. He never guilt-trips you. He tells you the truth, and he has*

penetrating insight. He is a wise man. One time when we were in college, I was freaking out about how I was going to bomb a test. He wisely reminded me that I deserved to bomb it since I hadn't studied. I could always count on Dick to not sugar coat anything. Weeks or months could go by without our talking to each other, but whenever we would speak there was never any hint of "why haven't you called me?" It's always been like we just spoke yesterday. Whenever we hang up with each other, each of us usually says, "I love you." I suppose for manly men like us that's pretty rare.

The 2 Most Important Words: "I'm sorry." There's an important difference between these two words and the six most important words: "I admit that I was wrong." What "I'm sorry" adds to the humility is compassion. We say "I'm sorry" when we make a mistake, but we also say it when we feel empathy for the suffering of another person, as in, "I'm sorry for the loss of your father" or, "I'm sorry you're feeling so bad."

It's important to say these two words within our families, but it's also important between friends. It affirms an emotional connection between two people that runs deeper than common interests, deeper than having a few laughs together. It connects heart to heart. Of course, it's extra important to say "I'm sorry" when you are the one who screwed up! But there is more going on here than some words to smooth things over.

By the way — don't neglect the flip side to this one: forgiveness. When a friend has screwed up and hurt you in some way, accept the apology graciously. Most people don't try to hurt us — especially our friends. It helps to make the most positive interpretation of our friends' actions and intentions that we can. And we might, if we are feeling especially generous, be proactive here by extending our forgiveness even without waiting for the "I'm sorry."

The 1 Least Important Word: "Me." It's not easy not thinking about ourselves. Most of our waking life is spent thinking about ourselves. The old saying, "I'm not much, but I'm all I think about" is an apt description of the human condition. It is a useful habit for our survival, but that's about all. Friendship requires putting others in front of ourselves. When people are courteous, they are thinking about others. Being thoughtful, being considerate, smiling, saying please and thank you, are all basic human niceties, but they are based on the understanding that there is someone other than ourselves who deserves our consideration.

Putting yourself second is a problem for some people — those who frequently put themselves last on the priority list and quietly resent it. But most of us do not have that problem; we have the opposite problem of putting ourselves first. The solution: **Cultivate selflessness.**

> *Several years ago I attended a week-long conference/retreat intended to offer participants ways of seeing and thinking*

that would help them professionally and personally. There were people from the helping professions: physicians, teachers and psychologists, as well as business leaders and attorneys. There were lectures, discussions, case studies and journal writing, but there were also ample opportunities for quiet thought and contemplation. It was during one of those quiet moments of reflection that I had a brilliant flash of insight that seemed at the time to be as profound as the discovery of the theory of relativity. Ready for the gem?

*Much of what people experience as unhappiness has at its root **selfishness.** I want. I want. I want. I want more. I want a better one. I want a different one. I want a shiny red one. I want a better position. I want more attention. I want less attention. Why can't I get what I want? For the whole week, every time I was disappointed or irritated or pissed about something, it was because something didn't go my way. My insatiable desire for something or other was at the root of my pain. Granted, it wasn't physical pain, but emotional pain is still a drag.*

It's easy to see my kids have the same reaction to not getting what they want. They might whine or throw a tantrum when this happens. We adults just hide it better. Greg shared with me a similar insight from AA. Some people see the glass as half empty. Some people see the glass as half full. Some people couldn't care less: they just want a bigger glass. **Our job is to constantly see and challenge our own selfishness.**

What Goes Around

Being good with people is something we work at for our whole life. It's as simple as eating healthily, exercising regularly, and getting a good night's sleep. It's not rocket science — it's obvious. Yet it does requires effort. If you have good friends already, nurture those precious relationships to keep them strong. If you are happy and fulfilled with your work, your family, and everything else that fills your day, and you don't seem to have a need for close friendships, that's fine. Just be pleasant and friendly to whomever you encounter, and be open to growing into a deeper level of friendship when the time is right.

> *A friend just told me of one of the principles he tries to live by with varying degrees of success. He said that friends will come and go but enemies accumulate. People have long memories. Avoid making enemies if you can avoid it, they tend to want to get you back.*

Secrets of the Obvious

- Be good company, and keep good company

- Cultivate your important friendships outside work and family

- Say what you mean, mean what you say, and don't say it meanly

- Ask people what they think and listen to what they say

- Show your gratitude and appreciation

- Challenge your own selfishness

Chapter 7

Health at Work

I really respect Ennis, a man whose job for the past 6 years has been to single-handedly keep a 28,000-square-foot training facility clean. Over 200,000 people have used the facility over those years. He has been called upon to clean up after all of us. The place looks as good as it does because of him, but I'm not impressed with him because he does such a great job. I'm impressed with how he goes about his job. I am not exaggerating to say that I have never seen Ennis complain about anything he has to do. And some of the stuff he has had to clean up I won't go into. He does it with such levelheaded professionalism and positive attitude you'd think he loved being a janitor. The truth is, I have never asked him how he feels about his job. I'm sure it's mixed, but the way he handles himself is a testimony to his wisdom about work. Ask anyone who knows him. He is remarkable.

After I wrote this I asked Ennis why he seemed so happy in doing his job. He said that it was from his mom. She always raised him to have the attitude that you should be happy no matter what job you do. If you don't like what you do, do something else. Don't you love it when moms are wise?

Love It or Leave It

It's obvious how we can create a healthy and balanced life at work that becomes a source of energy, meaning and pleasure rather than a being an annoying drag on our lives. All we need to do is follow George Burns's advice: **"Fall in love with what you do for a living, and you'll never have to work a day in your life."** Maybe it's not so obvious or easy to do, or else we would see more coffee mugs in the office reading TGIM instead of TGIF.

It is possible to love your job, but like all the other areas of health, it requires discipline and a little effort. OK — for some people with some jobs, it takes a lot of effort. It's just easier to complain about our work — either inwardly or, worse, outwardly to everyone around us. Just like pigging out or disregarding your friends, complaining about your work or having a job you hate really sucks energy from your life in ways that don't show up right away.

I was sitting in a doctor's office waiting room writing this when I asked a rather chatty and friendly receptionist what she liked about her job. She replied, "Leaving at the end of the day."

The challenge for all of us is to treat our work with reverence and respect. Our work is much more than a means of making some money to buy stuff, or a way to pass the time or get to the weekend. It is what we spend the majority of our life doing, and so why not do it in such a way that it adds energy to our lives? And if that's impossible, then find another job.

> *My wife had a job she was initially excited about, but after a while it became increasingly clear that it wasn't a good fit for her. After the initial honeymoon, she was so depleted by her experience that if you asked her how was work today the response was always a sigh followed by the noncommittal, "OK, I guess." Jan isn't the type to complain outwardly, but it was obvious to me what a drag it was for her.*
>
> *When she finally left, her spirits rose immediately. In her case the wise thing to do was to leave. You could argue that it is more courageous to stick it out and try to change the work environment, but that's up to each person. She clearly made the right call. The work she's doing now she absolutely loves.*

So maybe the answer is a combination of **"find the job you love"** and **"love the job you find."**

Loving your job does require effort. That may seem counterintuitive since you may be thinking, "Why should

I have to work at loving my job? If I have a great job, it shouldn't be so hard." Wrongo! No matter what the job, there are always aspects of it that are less pleasant or that outright stink. The key is to deal with that stuff the way you deal with anything unpleasant. Just do it. Don't blow it out of proportion. Don't dwell on it. And don't let it become the bulk of what you do. Whether you're self employed or work for a company, do the scut work part of your job quickly. It's just like washing the dishes, changing diapers, or taking out the garbage — not fun but necessary. There is no job that doesn't have some BS attached.

I worked with dozens of professional facilitators, consultants, and speakers when I was working in the above-mentioned conference center. We worked as a team putting on 3½-day conferences for management teams from around the country. Since I was always there and the rest of the team would change composition, I could observe how different people would assume their roles and responsibilities as they rotated through the center.

Their roles were usually in some level of support. Certain people radiated gratitude for their opportunity to help out, even though they weren't in a central role. Others would grouse around, going through the motions of being there. One woman stood out: Katie. When she started, she was clearly over her head, but she set as a goal to become one of the core team. What she lacked in skill she made up in attitude and effort. This was a woman who, like Ennis, never complained, would do whatever the team needed, and always had an incredibly positive attitude. She kept working until she was 8½ months pregnant but never backed away from anything that needed to get done, ever. No sighs, no eyeball rolls, no malicious obedience. She just did it. She loves what she does and it shows. She came back to work after her two kids were born. It's no coincidence that she has become one of the most appreciated and valued members of our team.

Have you ever noticed how two people doing the exact same job can have a completely different experience? It doesn't matter what the job is. I travel a lot, so the experience that blows my mind is the airline ticket counter person or the gate agent. Now, clearly this is a stressful, highly demanding job. Why is it that some people are incredibly friendly, service- oriented, smiling, and problem solving, while the person right next to them is sour, bitter, angry and bothered by having to deal with you? They have the same job!

A tale of two gate agents: "I'm sorry first class is full, but I can put you in an exit row. Wait here in the gate area — you never know when someone might not show for first class. We may be able to get you a seat. Let's hope (with an encouraging smile)." Versus: "First is full, take your assigned seat please (with the standard-issue blank stare)." Southwest Airlines has a hiring policy that looks for people with great attitudes — being good with people and passionate about their work. They can train those people later to have the right skills. I don't know for sure, but I'm willing to bet that the first gate agent is someone who loves her job.

Sometimes I'm unaware of how I'm approaching my work. I'll think that I can't wait until the weekend, or an upcoming vacation. I'll say things like, "I have to go to work today. I've got a ton of garbage to deal with." Or sometimes you hear people saying, "Thank God it's Friday" or "Wednesday is Hump day." Just like a rambunctious kid who needs to be settled down. Remind yourself how you are disrespecting your work when you say that stuff. If you don't like your job for all kinds of legitimate reasons, find another job or change your attitude about your current situation. Change the aspects of your job that need changing. Don't tolerate your job like a bad marriage you stay in for the sake of the kids. **Fix it or leave.** Don't bitch about it.

Here are some ideas about how to fix it.

Your Unique Abilities

My friend and colleague Bert Whitehead, a gifted financial planner, divides our work lives into four categories:

1. ***I'm Incompetent:*** There are parts of our jobs at which we are really incompetent. If these tasks are a large part of our jobs, then we probably should find another line of work. But all jobs have something in them that makes us fumble and sweat. It might be public speaking, or writing, or keeping track of details, or budget planning, or fixing the copy machine. Come to think of it, there are potentially a huge number of areas where people can be incompetent. For me, there are too many to name, but at the top of the list are technology, anything mechanical, organizing complex data into manageable tasks, and keeping track of paperwork. There is a colleague at work who knows me well. As soon as I write some notes for a future presentation, she'll grab them and file them before I lose them.

   The best thing to do is to delegate as many of these tasks as possible without becoming an irresponsible jerk. **Sometimes we just have to suck it up and do these things the best we can.** Some stuff you might be able to ignore, but that can catch up with you. Like maybe you are not good at doing the record keeping needed for your taxes. That's dangerous to ignore, so delegate it if you can. My assistant, Jo, is an absolute godsend when it comes to helping me keep track of records. And if that's not an option, then just do it the best you can and get it over with, if possible without listening to that destructive voice inside you that says, "I stink at this, so I hate it." Just keep quiet and do it.

There is always a learning curve when it comes to our jobs so there will be a time when we will be incompetent. If that period takes 10 years to change, we've got a problem. My friend, the chairman of a medical school department, told me he spent most of his career hoping no one would find out he was incompetent. He was exaggerating, of course, but I think many people spend a lot of their work lives trying to convince people that they know what they are doing. Let's face it — plenty of people are in the wrong line of work or the wrong job

2. ***I'm Competent Enough:*** There are parts of your job at which you are competent. You can do them well enough. I can write a decent business letter. It won't be a great letter and I don't get a lot of pleasure out of doing it, but I can do it OK. If you don't find a lot of what you do on your job at least in this category, then you are probably going to be miserable.

3. ***I'm Excellent:*** There are those things at which you are truly excellent. You know this because people tell you so, and you know it because you just feel it. People have hired you because of it, and they will continue to do so. For me, it's public speaking or facilitating a certain type of meeting. I work hard at it, my audiences appreciate my work, people pay me well to do it, and I derive a lot of satisfaction from it.

4. ***I'm Uniquely Gifted:*** And finally, there are
those things at which you are uniquely gifted:
talents and skills that you alone have. I'm not
saying that you have to be Einstein or Picasso
here, but on the other hand, you probably are the
Picasso of something. Maybe it's dealing with
troubled colleagues or customers. Maybe it's
handling time pressure, or coming up with off-
the-wall creativity, or making a new person feel
welcome. Maybe it's looking after details or doing
the all-important follow-through on a project. Or
helping your team to prioritize. For some people
their unique talent is selling. **The secret here is
to discover what those things are, and then
to organize your work life around that
ability.** Find ways to do those things regularly as
part of your contribution to your organization and
to the world.

The obvious secret here is to find ways to shift your work
from category #1 toward the higher categories. Bert
Whitehead suggests that you should spend no more than
15% of your day working with your incompetencies, and
no more than 30% with tasks at which you are merely
competent. Now, I know you are thinking that it's
impossible to break down how you spend your time in
such a way that you could allocate numerical
percentages to various activities. But the goal is that you
think consciously about how you spend your time. **Are
you doing stuff that you really shouldn't be doing?**
A gifted surgeon, like my friend Mark, should definitely
not be spending his time dealing with insurance
agencies. He should be talking to patients or operating

on them. Granted, he needs to know what his staff has to deal with, but his time is much better spent with patients and their families.

You might well argue that many people work at jobs where they do not have the power to shift their work around that way because they have to do what they are told. True — though you might have more freedom than you think, especially if you can negotiate with your supervisor about your job. Even if you can't negotiate with your boss, do whatever you can in your job to maximize your unique talents. Make this shift to the extent that you can. And by the way — if you are a supervisor or leader who wants to attract and retain employees, then you might want to engage in such a conversation so you can find ways to help people do what they do best. This is what Jim Collins, in his book *Good to Great,* means by getting the right people in the right seats on the bus. Including you. **Your job is to be a great coach.**

Good at Something

One of the obvious but nonetheless valuable things my father told me was to have a marketable skill. What he meant was, have a skill that, no matter what happens, you can always earn a living. In the real world, this might also mean getting the credentials to demonstrate that you have that skill. A simple example: Having a college degree will open a lot of doors for you. Yes, we know the stories of how Tom Monaghan created his Domino's Pizza empire without virtue of his degree, and Bill Gates was a college dropout. But these people are the exceptions — that's why their stories are so compelling. You need to get into the game. And to do that, you probably need to pay the ante.

In my case, the ante was a Ph.D. degree. I had learned a lot as an undergraduate and even more earning my masters. I knew enough to be helpful to people and I also knew that every experience I had with clients would increase my knowledge and my value to future clients. But that was not good enough.

In the world in which I wanted to live and work, the Ph.D. carries a lot of weight. The doctorate means a lot to people I wanted to work with and for. I did not think doing the research and writing the dissertation would cause me to learn a lot that would be especially useful to me in my work with private clients and organizations. I was not interested in being a research psychologist, and I was not looking to work at a university. But the Ph.D. means something in the minds of others, and it was therefore an extremely useful credential. As it turns out, the process of getting my doctorate was valuable because of the discipline I learned, the people I met, and the content I discovered. But I didn't know that in advance, and it would have been worth doing even without all those

*benefits. The main value of the Ph.D. was
that it makes people think you are smart.
It's an accomplishment that has some
inherent value. People will pay you more
just because you have it. The fact that my
Mom and Dad used to introduce me as Dr.
Harry Cohen was also a kick for them.*

**In the job setting we have a similar opportunity to
learn a marketable skill.** There may not be a degree
involved, but there will be something that will make you
stand out from the crowd. Remember, the idea is to find
a way for you to move up from doing those things at
which you are merely competent to those at which you
are excellent or uniquely gifted. Obviously, it's easier to
do this if you have an area of excellence or a unique gift.
Learn about the new technology that your company will
be implementing. Get the extra degree. Take the
overseas assignment. Learn the language. Become the
expert on the matrix organization, or modular scheduling,
or the new accounting procedure, or anything that will
benefit you or your organization in the long run. And if
you get some tangible credentials from the experience,
all the better. Let folks know. Becoming a certified
master technician in the automotive world means you are
capable of negotiating higher pay, benefits, and more
flexibility than if you are merely a great technician. A
gifted carpenter with his own tools will have job security
for life regardless of the ups and downs in the economy.
The same is true in any profession or craft.

*My sister earned a law degree that she
used for only a short time because she*

146

became a stay-at-home mom. After about nine years, she easily re-entered the work force with degree in hand. She got a job as a lawyer that she actually likes. She is currently a magistrate and poised to make some career moves that will earn her even more money and freedom. The fact that she's smart and finished her undergraduate degree at Penn in three years doesn't matter. Her credential is what allows her to earn.

Your Brand

This idea may sound a bit shallow when you first read it. I know — let's all turn ourselves into a brand of soft drinks or breakfast cereals so that we can sell ourselves. Selling ourselves does not mean duping people into buying us. We're branding ourselves all the time. My brother-in-law is a partner in a small law firm. You would never think of him as selling himself. He's too modest and humble. The truth is, he is as successful as he is because of his personal brand. His reputation is one of the most honest, selfless, and straightforward men in his community.

Becoming conscious of your brand means presenting yourself in a way that is **consistent**, **credible**, and **clear**. It means being all these things with regard to who you are. It means delivering on a promise. People with whom you interact at work are, in a sense, buying a package of stuff. That stuff is you — who you are, what you do, and how you do it. This is true if you are an independent contractor who is dealing with clients — looking for new ones or working with established ones — or a member of a larger organization — looking to work on exciting projects that will enhance your career. People want to know: What does he bring to the party? Do we want him on our team? Will he represent us or our company well? What is his reputation? Should we promote her? Should we invite her to the meeting? What do we get by hiring him? What are this guy's values?

Your brand is not something you can fake. As a species, we have evolved with highly sensitive insincerity detectors, so people can see through the BS and spot a phony. We know how to spot the fake smile and it makes us cringe. **There's no such thing as a "hidden agenda."** The only way to be **credible** is to be honest about who you are and what you stand for.

Be true to your values — that's where being **consistent** comes in. Your behavior needs to flow from what you believe in. If your reputation is that of a person who cares passionately about his work, then it will show in your behavior consistently. It's not about doing a slick sales job with you as the product. It's about integrity. **If someone asks you in a job interview about you, all you have to do is tell the truth.** Describe what you do well and what you are lousy at doing. They'll find out eventually. If you're self-employed, tell your prospective clients exactly what they will get by hiring you. Also tell them what they won't get.

What we can learn from the marketers is about being **clear**. If your brand image is the person who is great at getting people to work together, or great at seeing the big picture, or looking after the details, or working with data, or doing research, or intuitively sensing what the customers want, or analyzing complex problems, or speaking to groups — whatever it is, present yourself that way so that people know what value you are adding to any project. No, I'm not saying you have to do a song and dance or create an infomercial. What I am saying **the essence of who you are and what you do should be crystal clear to you and anybody else.**

People should know what they're getting and not getting when they hire you. When people came in to see me as a therapist to decide if they really wanted to keep seeing me, they sized me up. What is his approach? What is he going to do for us? If I were not clear about who I was and what I would offer them, I'd never see them again. By the same token, if I were crystal clear about who I was and how I did therapy, they'd say this either is or is not the brand of therapy we want. That's the way it should be. The same is true now with corporate clients. I got a call to work with an executive team that was basically a dysfunctional family. The guy who called was the CFO of the organization. He knew what he was asking for; he knew what he would get.

When my wife and I were looking for a builder to build our new home, we did the usual asking around for recommendations and then got bids from several builders. The choice we made was based not only on the impression he made with us but also his reputation. His brand was honesty, quality, and pleasantness.

An executive who was recently promoted brought together her whole organization to tell them who she was, what she was about, what she expected, and what were her values. She didn't tell them, "this is my brand," but in effect she told them just that. She wasn't selling them on the package — she was informing them of what her promise was to them. If she delivers on that promise, her brand will be clear, consistent and credible.

Another man was promoted to vice president who was completely apolitical. He didn't care who in senior management he irritated if it meant telling the truth. His reputation was that of a brilliant man who cared about his people but was never afraid to say that the emperor had no clothes. Besides a great wit, he has an incredible ability to cut through the BS. He was passed over for promotion so many times that people thought that his brand of leadership was not valued in this company. When he got the promotion a lot of people called him to say, "It's about time."

Our reputation at work is extremely valuable. In fact, it's priceless. Remember that. **Everything we do in our work creates an overall impression of who we are.** That's the good news and the bad. We're either enhancing and polishing our brand, or we're sullying it. Nothing is ever neutral. People are hired and fired, promoted and demoted because of their reputation. The good stuff they do follows them; so does the bad. You know the expression, "You are what you eat." You can add another one, "You are what you have done."

Problems and Challenges

What's the difference between a problem and a challenge? Actually, it may be helpful to see the issue in terms of three ways.

Annoyance — When you are being annoyed, what you are experiencing is the fact that something is rubbing you the wrong way. You are being hassled, and it makes you angry or stressed. Recall that great employee I dealt with at the Northwest Airlines ticket counter. What if, instead, I encountered someone who perceived my difficulty as a pain in her day? Not only would my flight plans be screwed up, but she probably would have had a joyless experience as well, one where her main achievement would be to have had me go away mad or disappointed while she felt like the victim for having to deal with someone like me. Everybody loses.

Problem — It's a big step forward to be able to transform our annoyances into problems. Why? Because problems have solutions. OK, so they don't all have solutions — at least not yet. But my point is that when you see the annoyance as a problem, you start moving toward a solution. There is a process under way, and that's a step in the right direction. Your whole attitude changes to one of constructive action. Fix it. Solve it. Deal with it.

151

Challenge — Now it gets personal. When we see a problem as a challenge, we become invested in finding a positive outcome. We become committed, and there's an intrinsic reward involved. We may see this as an opportunity for growth. Let's say, for example, that your computer gets a virus. (If this hasn't yet happened to you, it will. Trust me on this.) Now, if dealing with computers is an area of your incompetence, then call for your computer person. But if that's not an option for you, move as quickly as possible through the annoyance stage to where you see it as a problem for which you are seeking a solution. Run the out-of-date virus scan program that came with your computer. Figure out where and how to download and install a new one. That's problem-solving. It becomes a challenge when you see this as an opportunity to learn something more about computers and computer viruses. And if you are like me, you may also invent some new curse words in the process. By the way, if we don't back up everything on our computer that we want to save, we deserve to suffer.

This may seem simplistic, and it is. Sometimes we do well to leave it at the problem level so we don't feel so bad when we are stumped. Time to delegate without taking it personally. Sorry, but I don't trust myself to do my own income taxes, and I don't at all feel like a failure when I admit it. In fact, it makes me feel smart to recognize this limitation. And very often it's enormously productive and satisfying to transform a large annoying feeling or an overwhelming situation into a clearly defined problem or, more likely, a series of problems.

152

This puts it into the Manageable Zone, where we can go to work on it.

So what I'm really saying is that whether we see problems as challenges that we welcome as opportunities for personal growth and satisfaction, or as annoyances that ruin the tranquility of your day — the choice is up to *us*. As I said earlier, **we can't always control what life dumps on our plate, but we can control our attitude toward it.**

> *I'm sure you know a million stories about people who have dealt with tough challenges at work. Recently a good friend was laid off from his work. He has two small children and very little savings. His wife is on medical disability from her job. What he told me is that he doesn't have the luxury of getting depressed about his circumstance. He immediately laid out a plan of attack. What it has forced him to do is get organized, get assertive, and get some work. He has landed several pieces of work as a freelance contractor and has some prospects cooking. What is impressive about him is how disciplined he is. I have no doubt he will succeed. He also has a great sense of humor. He told me he's learned to take rejection quite well. He quoted the fictional character, Bob, the motivational speaker from a recently canceled sitcom, "No is only yes to a different question."*

There is a basic rule of all challenges at work: There is only one way to deal with any difficulty at work and that is to go through it. Not around it. If you're staring at a mountain of paperwork or a huge project, the healthiest way to approach it is one shovel at a time. It doesn't matter how big the pile is or what the pile is made of. All of us have had to shovel dung. **One shovel at a time and you will get through it.** People say, "How can you write a book?" It's actually quite daunting, if I think about the whole thing. But if I just focus on the chapter, or even the simple point I'm trying to make, it just goes. One shovel at a time. One chapter at a time. One patient at a time. One project at a time. When we were climbing up Mt. Rainier, there was this endless series of slow steps, one at a time, up the mountain. It felt incredibly monotonous, but the payoff was worth it. The same is true in every task we take on. As my Dad said, "Procrastination is the thief of time." Just do it now.

Meaning in Your Work

This may sound a bit corny, but it's not. **Treat your work with reverence.** Any kind of work can be seen as "holy work" — it's all a matter of attitude. I'm sure that Ennis, the janitor at our conference center, has found that kind of meaning in his work, as has this woman at the Northwest Airlines counter:

> *I went to the Northwest counter at Detroit Metro Airport and discovered a problem with my ticket. My connecting flight no longer existed, and it appeared that I*

could not get to Los Angeles on time to meet my client. The woman I spoke with there was totally involved in helping me solve my problem. She was cheerful and confident that she could come up with something, and she did, trying one thing after another on her computer until she said, "Bingo! This will do it!" But what's important to me now is that she clearly saw that her job is to make a difference in the world. She contributed significantly to my happiness by solving one customer's problem. I thanked her for her efforts, and she obviously enjoyed the whole process. She was finding meaning in her work. Her job wasn't ticket agent, it was solving problems for people. And I know from very different experiences in dealing with other people in similar jobs that the key here is in her attitude — not in the job itself.

It's a matter of attitude, and to a large extent, you are in total control of your attitude. **Don't complain about your work, because if you talk about it in negative terms, it will become what you say it is.** And this means that you should not hang out with people who enjoy complaining about their jobs, for their attitudes can be infectious. You know how it works.

David Stringer, a writer who helped me edit this book, says he has four criteria for accepting a new writing assignment:

- Can I do a great job?
- Will I enjoy the person I work with?
- Will I learn something?
- Will I be adding value to the world?

(Dave doesn't usually mention his fifth question: Do I need the money?)

Adding value to the world is important for him, and it should be. He agreed to work with me because he really felt that the book would help people lead better lives. He does work with corporate clients, not because his work will help them make more money — though he hopes it will — but because it will help the people in the organization work better on teams, or treat one another fairly and constructively. **Whatever your work is, you can find meaning in it if you can see how you are adding value to the world.** It doesn't have to be the whole world — just the corner of it where you operate. Look for that value and meaning.

Over the years, I have worked with thousands of dealership management teams and Ford Motor Company managers. In all that time, it has been remarkable how many employees of those managers have shared with me how certain bosses were such a positive influence in their lives. **These managers were much more than good bosses or good leaders, they were and are inspirations to the people who work for them.** When people would tell me how their boss was as important to them as a great coach or even a great parent, I would usually ask them if they told the boss that. They would usually say no. As Kahil Gibran said, **"Work is love made manifest."**

A Culture of Excellence

Many books have been written lately about how to create an organizational culture. Most of them describe the task as something that leaders are supposed to do — by creating reward systems, engineering the structure and processes, highlighting the history and heroes of the organization, and by choosing language carefully in order to reflect deep assumptions about how things are to be done. All this is very well and good, especially if you are the CEO. But what about the rest of us?

You don't have to be the "big boss" in order to create a culture of excellence. Organizational psychologists, consultants and effective leaders today recognize that everyone in an organization exercises leadership. Everyone. We don't all decide whether to bring out a new product, downsize the company, or merge with the neighborhood conglomerate. But we do all exercise an influence over the climate of the people we work with. And we work happier — and more effectively — if that climate is positive, and if it values excellence.

How do we do it?

- Celebrate small successes — our own and those of our colleagues. Part of your culture can be to do this regularly. And don't wait until you win the Super Bowl in order to celebrate. Finishing an

157

unpleasant task, meeting a deadline, having a good conversation with a client, getting rid of a destructive client, completing a portion of a project — any of these is worth a small celebration, for yourself and for your team.

- See how what you and your team are doing makes a difference — that you are contributing to something worthwhile. Articulate this to yourself and to one another. If you can't do this, then you might consider looking for a different job.

- Don't hang out with people who drag you down, belittling the work you do together. You might even want to speak up to such people to try to change the tone of the conversation. This is a form of leadership.

- Recognize what it feels like to take joy in your work. You all know the feeling: It's just fun doing this, and they even pay you to do it! Time flies by, and when you come home at the end of the day, you're tired and energized at the same time. We need to stop to acknowledge when this is happening, and to understand that it usually happens when we are working well, using our unique talents on a meaningful project.

The most important thing is never to be satisfied with a level of mediocrity in your work world. Challenge yourself and others to continually raise the bar in whatever way is feasible. Some of us can get quite comfortable with a merely adequate level of performance. You know the expression, "Good enough for government work." Doesn't it blow your mind when you see some organization run as if excellence were the furthest thing from their mind? I once went through a check-out line at a local sporting goods store where the entire organization has spent years perfecting the culture of inefficiency and ineptitude. When the guy handed me my change, I said, "A thank you would be nice." He replied, "It's on the receipt."

> *Last week I bought a laptop. Four different people helped me, and each one represented the four levels of performance. The first one was so nonchalant that it seemed as if he weren't even there. He couldn't have cared less about the customer, the product, or himself for that matter. He looked like a total slob. I think he probably wandered into that department by mistake. The second guy was a little more competent, but just barely. He certainly took his job more seriously, and yet he gave completely incorrect information. The third guy loved his job and computers, and he was also a great salesman. The fourth guy was even more gifted than the third. Not only did he love his job, people were lining up to talk to him and ask him questions. He actually told me to get a different computer at a different store because it would fit my needs better.*

Look around you where you work and challenge sloppiness. Sometimes we can get so used to it that it seems normal. Here's an obvious tip: **Start with yourself.**

Get Organized

One of the most obvious things you can do to waste less time, get more done and feel more satisfied with what you do with your life is to become conscious and deliberate about how you spend your time. **Work is one of those things where *other* people can determine your schedule, if you let them.** Obviously there are plenty of things that you can't control in terms of how you spend your time. But there are tons of things that we can decide are important or not, urgent or not. Steven Covey wrote a great book about time management called *First Things First.* The point of the book is that everything we do falls into one of four categories:

1. Important and urgent
2. Important but not urgent
3. Not important but urgent
4. Not important and not urgent

In order to be effective with the use of our time, we have to understand how what we are doing falls into one of those four areas. In fact, all you have to do is focus on just one, the important stuff. **The secret is to do the important but not urgent stuff first, since we are more likely to procrastinate those things that can be put off.** The urgent stuff will always grab our attention and demand our time. It's the important stuff that we really need to focus on. Exercise, goal setting, planning your day, calling a prospective client, cleaning up a mess at work, calling an old friend, finishing this chapter, are all things that are very important but could wait until later. Urgent and important stuff are the crises that require you to respond immediately.

The real culprits in our day are the not important things, regardless of whether they are urgent or not. Phone calls that you don't have to take, busy work, stuff someone else should do, waste-of-time meetings, conversations that have no value, reading something that you don't need to read — these all are time-killers. Taking five or ten minutes to plan your day, either the night before or in the morning, is one of the simplest ways to get more organized. **Write down the one or two important things you would like to accomplish in your day.** If you get those things done, your day will be more successful than if you accomplish 10 things on your to-do list, but they are all unimportant things. **Just remember to focus on the most important stuff, and everything else will eventually get done by you or someone else.** Don't make yourself crazy.

Another way to think about this is in terms of the difference between being **efficient** and being **effective**. The goal is to be effective by choosing to spend your time doing things that will make a difference. You know you can be incredibly efficient doing tons of things that don't really matter one bit. People are impressed with their ability to multitask. That's just a fancy way of doing lots of things at once. Big deal. What you should do is fewer things that make a difference. **Nobody cares how busy you are except you.**

If you think about the days at work when you felt the most effective, successful and energized, it was usually because you got something important accomplished. That was no accident. **Proper planning will usually prevent poor performance.** Effective carpenters always organize their toolbox. I know it's boring and you already know it, that's OK. Do it anyway. **Measure twice, cut once.**

A friend of mine is an executive in large company. He recently asked his senior managers what is the first thing they do in the morning when they come into work. They all replied that they check their e-mails. "Checking your email," he told them, "is probably the least important task you will perform all day." **The most important thing they should do?** His answer: **"Say good morning to your people and find out what is going on in their lives."** If his managers do it properly, they will – in just a few minutes – build their team, find out critical information, and demonstrate genuine leadership. He is one of those rare execs that is both competent and wise.

Make Your Own Lunch

> *The other day someone said to me, "Wow, you really love what you do, don't you?" In that moment I loved my job. I suspect he was thinking that I had the perfect job. I was speaking passionately to a group of*

*people about something I believe in. I was
thinking it makes a difference in the world;
I was doing it well, and people seemed to
appreciate the effort. But the truth is that I
struggle with the same stuff that everyone
struggles with. There is no perfect job. Am
I competent? How can I do this job even
better? Is this what I should be doing with
my life? What is the best use of my
talents? What am I going to be when I
grow up? Should I stay at this gig or move
on? Should I grow in a different direction?
Should I expand my business? Should I
take that job across town?*

The point of questioning your work life is to make certain
that you don't waste your time or your life doing
something that depletes you. **Your work life needs
renewal and rededication, just as much as your
marriage does.** Status quo may not be appropriate, for
you can change from being in a groove to being in a rut.

Just like good food or good friendship, your work should
give you a tremendous feeling of satisfaction and
gratitude for being able to contribute. **If your job
stinks, change it.** Don't become victimized by work that
isn't healthy for you.

There is an old joke about a guy who constantly
complains about what he gets for lunch every day. When
he opens his lunch box, it's always the same thing, ham
and cheese. After hearing this guy complain constantly,
his colleague says to him, "If you don't like ham and

cheese, why don't you ask your wife to make something different for you?" He replies, "What are you talking about? I make my own lunch."

Secrets of the Obvious

- Find a job you love, or learn to love the job you find

- Cultivate your brand

- Turn annoyances into problems, problems into challenges

- Appreciate how what you do makes a difference

- Organize your work time so you give priority to the important stuff

- Make your own lunch

Chapter 8

Family Health

My sister has three daughters. She and her husband have been married for 30 years. Watching each of them grow up has taught me a lot. There were times during the kids' teen years that none of us ever thought they would get through. What has been so cool to watch is how they have not just survived, but thrived. One daughter is in medical school, one daughter is becoming a teacher, and the other is running the alumni office at the school from which she graduated. It 's not just that they have turned out well, it's that they are truly confident, sweet and considerate young women. It was not luck that got them through. Patty and Warren never gave up. They have a rule in their family that after two years the statute of limitations runs out on getting into trouble for deeds committed long ago. They have enough trust now to have great fun talking about some of the shenanigans the kids pulled years ago. Some of those stunts the kids have shared with me, and I'll never tell my sister. I hope I can laugh in the same way with my boys one day

Everybody has a family, and each family is unique. And no family is perfect. But just as with everything else in life, there are certain rules that apply to family life that will make it easier to experience your family as a tremendous source of joy and energy rather than an enormous hassle or worse.

As a therapist, I often give families and couples advice about what they should and shouldn't do to keep their families healthy. A wise mentor, one of my professors, once told me that he would never go to a therapist who wasn't as old as he was since a younger therapist would be less likely to fully understand the dynamics of the family: they hadn't lived it. Many of my clients would say to me half jokingly that they couldn't wait to see how my kids turn out, since I was such an expert when it came to their kids. Well, I certainly don't claim to be an authority on the subject of family. There are far wiser and more experienced people in the world who have managed to raise and keep their families healthy. All I can offer are a few tips on how not to make a mess of our very fragile family life. I think they are obvious, useful, and practiced by millions of families including my own with varying degrees of success.

Marriage

Say It and Show It

People get a kick out of my advising them not to put their marriage on the "no maintenance" setting. You know how that one goes: **"I told you I loved you**

when we got married — if it changes, I'll let you know." Most people don't do enough to consciously maintain the quality of their marriage. They let a million things take priority over the sanctity of the marriage — kids, work, house, money, or whatever. They take their spouse for granted — an almost guaranteed way to tick off a husband or wife. They don't do anything romantic. Instead, they assume that the spouse will be there because they have so much history. And then they are also incredibly surprised when the spouse wants to split. "I don't understand what went wrong. We were together for so many years."

Well, here's a news flash: **You don't get credit for years married.** It's not like equity in your house, or years that qualify for retirement. The years of your marriage mean only one thing — you've been married that long. The real point is the quality of your marriage. If you don't tell, show, demonstrate, and do stuff for your mate — stuff that really signals to him or her your love and respect, then you're headed for one of those classic conversations with a lawyer. "I don't know why she wasn't happy. I was always a good provider. I never fooled around. I was never violent. I didn't go out with the guys." These days that is not good enough — nor should it be.

The bottom line is this: Those demonstrations of how much you love your mate are not the only things keeping a marriage in good shape, but they are among the most important. **Let your spouse know how much you appreciate him or her — a LOT!** Oh, and one more thing: Do it in a way that they would appreciate. Some people want flowers, some people want words, some people want action, some people want stuff, some people want physical touch, some people want help with the housework, yard work, or cooking. Find out who you are married to, what they want, how and when they want it. Then do it. And if you think you do a great job already in this department, ask your spouse.

Don't Screw Around

The next most important thing to remember about keeping your marriage strong is so obvious that it amazes me that I have to talk about it. Here it is: Do not screw around with anyone but your spouse. I repeat — do not have sex with anyone but your spouse. That means no kissing, no fondling, no petting, no cyber-nookie, and no nothing. Clinton's escapades have now made it obvious to everyone that he was not the first nor will he be the last married person to quibble about what constitutes infidelity. "Yeah, but all we did was make out, we didn't have sex." People often say that when someone has an affair, it's not really about sex. I have news for you: Yes it is. Of course it's about trust, betrayal, honesty, intimacy, and that good old standby, lack of communication. But it's also about sex.

> *I once had a client who came to see me for marital therapy. After a couple of sessions with him and his wife, I suggested we meet alone. We went out for lunch and I convinced him that I would not tell his wife, but he had to come clean and tell me what was going on. He finally*

admitted to having an affair with someone at work. I told him point blank that he could either stay married or get divorced — I couldn't care less. He would have to decide that. What he could not do is stay married while continuing his affair. I explained to him that it would destroy his marriage if he continued. He said that no one had ever told him that. I wonder which people he had been talking to. I suppose there are plenty of therapists who would continue to work with a couple while one of them is screwing around; I'm not one of them. He did stop the affair and is currently happily married.

By the way, affairs don't just happen. They go from thought to word to deed. One of my favorite lines was "I didn't plan on it happening — it just happened." No it didn't. It's not like getting hit by a meteor that falls from the sky. You created it when you decided to flirt with him at the office party. You created it when you met for a drink after work. You created it when you went to her room on a business trip. You created it when you shared your feelings about how your marriage is not as great as it once was. Finally, you created it when you said to yourself, "What the hell, it's just a kiss." One more thing to remember about affairs: They occur because the person having the affair decided to.

Respect Boundaries

This brings up the issue of boundaries. Boundaries are the invisible lines between people through which we decide to allow information, people or things to pass — or not. **Healthy boundaries are an essential requirement of a great marriage.** There are some things that a couple should never allow to penetrate the boundary that encircles them. Another person's sexual organ is an example of that. By the same token, the couple's personal problems or intimate exchanges should not be shared with others. That stuff is no one's business. If you are having a serious problem with your partner, don't discuss it with other people who will make it worse. A friend has a daughter whose marriage is being poisoned by a little husband-bashing club that she hangs out with once a week. The boundaries between the couple should be permeable, but not so mushy that everything that one spouse experiences, the other should also. That is why there are doors on bathrooms and bedrooms. Some couples don't understand that. I often told clients that if you have a sexual dream about someone other than your spouse, you should not share it, no matter how interesting it seems to you. **Some information you should keep to yourself.**

Set High Standards

Every single couple has fights, disagreements and differences of opinion on everything from small stuff to big stuff, from toothpaste to childrearing. **The secret to a long and happy marriage is to set your standard for a healthy partnership quite high.** What that means is not to allow your marriage to deteriorate into co-existence, where you merely tolerate each other. There is nothing wrong with fighting as long as the fights are in the service of getting your partnership back in order. If you find yourself fighting a lot without satisfactory resolution for both of you, go find a therapist immediately. Also, if you can't get out of blah co-existence with your spouse, go to a therapist immediately. A friend of mine has been complaining about his wife a lot. He recently said to me, "I knew when I married her she was Mrs. Right, I just didn't know her first name was Always." He is quite funny, but he could have the makings of a pretty serious mess on his hands.

You know what fighting looks like, but you may not be aware of the subtle poison of co-existence. When couples co-exist, they merely tolerate each other. They aren't overtly rude or disrespectful. They just take care of their responsibilities without a lot of concern for the other: "I make the money, you raise the kids." They pass like ships in the night. They sit on the couch and watch TV without talking about much of anything. They have sex, maybe, but it is mostly out of obligation. They feel like roommates, not intimates. "How was your day? Fine. How was yours? Fine. What's for dinner?" Co-existence is a common phenomenon for every relationship, but the danger is in letting it go on for too long. People start to check out of the marriage. People start to have affairs with their work, their kids, their hobbies, their buddies, or food, booze, or anything else that gives them a lift. Don't be stupid — go get some help. Or start talking.

Avoid Toxic Behavior

A University of Washington study described the **Four Horsemen of the Apocalypse of Marriage: Blame, Defensiveness, Contempt, and Indifference.** The toxic nature of these attitudes and behaviors is obvious, and so are the alternatives:

1. Rather than blaming, take some responsibility.
2. Rather than getting defensive, listen to the kernel of truth your partner is saying.
3. Rather than expressing your contempt, demonstrate respect, at all times.
4. Finally, rather than checking out and being indifferent, look for solutions to the problem.

These are common sense rules, but people don't follow them. The solutions may be obvious to see and state, but they are not so easy to put into practice.

When you see your marriage heading down any of these paths, grab the reins and pull it in another direction. **Do not try to change the personality of your mate.** You can request all kinds of things for your mate to do and not do, but you cannot make him or her into someone else. Remember that. **Oh, and by the way, those little nasty comments you think don't matter — they do**:

- "You're just like your mother/father."
- "You really should lose some weight."
- "Is that what you call cleaning the garage?"
- "Thanks for nothing."
- "I don't have an opinion."

- "They're your parents."
- "Try thinking first."
- "What didn't you understand?"
- "I'll say it again slower."
- "I already told you."
- "You are impossible."
- "What do I get out of this?"
- "I should have never married you."

When a marriage is working, it is one of the best things in the world for keeping you happy and healthy. When it's not working, it really stinks. I am incredibly grateful to be married to such a humble, sweet, smart, giving, non-bitchy, non-defensive, thoughtful and introspective wife. The fact that she's not crazy helps, too. The truth is, I don't tell her enough what I just wrote. No excuse.

Kids

I should start this section by saying that my wisdom is based on being a parent of 10-year-old twin boys, being a 47-year-old son of great parents, and counseling hundreds of families. In other words, I don't have a clue. But there are certain things that seem obvious that if we would just remember, they would make our lives a whole lot easier and more fulfilling. First of all, every kid is different. I know people say that, but, until I had fraternal twin boys, I didn't know how true it really was. Kids come out completely pre-wired already. Their temperament is, to a large extent, already formed. **Our job, as parents, is to not mess them up.** Get clear with your partner on what are the basics, and then try as best as you can to do what you **and** your spouse think is

173

right. **There are no cookie cutter answers on how to parent properly.** Every book you read will give you useful tips. Every other parent can give you advice and perspective as well. Parenting is an art. **The most important thing to remember about parenting is to never give up.**

Set Limits

Kids need discipline. They don't like it but they need it — just like sleep, food and water. As kids, we lack the internal mechanism that controls our wanting. That's why it's so important to internalize our parents' limit setting. Have you ever seen a grown adult who acts like a kid that no one said "no" to? **One of the measures of a great parent is the ability to set limits on what is acceptable behavior and what is not.** What we will allow, tolerate, or support and what we will not.

A friend of mine has two grown sons. They both have turned out quite remarkable at this point in their lives. Recently, I was telling them about this book and I asked one of the boys to tell me one thing, of all the things his parents did, that had an influence on his life. His father was in the room so he might have answered because he was there, but he said after thinking about it for a bit, "Discipline. They really taught me the importance of discipline." The fact that he is a 4.0 student at Michigan is somewhat testimony to the truth of his response. I watched both kids growing up and I have to admit, I thought his Dad was a bit of a drill sergeant some times, but he was right. The fact is, his parents did a fabulous job. He told me recently that too many parents make the mistake of trying to be friends with their kids before realizing that their job is to be a parent first and a friend second.

There are a million ways to set limits, from curfews to TV time. **The point is to care less about how angry your kid will be for setting the limit, and to care more about what is right for the kid.** One of our neighbors has four kids, ages 9, 12, 16, and 19. They struggle like all parents to do the right thing; but they are great at setting limits for all their kids to internalize. When the 9-year-old comes over to play, he announces to us that his mom doesn't want him to play on the computer or Nintendo so he will have to do something else. Music to our ears.

Clarify Values

The simplest way to clarify values is to mean what you say, say what you mean, and don't say it meanly. You know what is important to you. You know how you want your kids to behave. You know what are the few values that you really want your kids to understand and live by. For Jan and me, there are a few basic ones. These are not in any order of priority:

- Be respectful of others.
- Be responsible.
- Contribute to the world.
- Take good care of yourself and your family.
- Do the right thing.

I'm sure there are more if I think of them, but these are the basics. **Our job as parents is to remind them of these basic values about nine million times.** Don't worry about sounding like a broken record — you do. I can still hear my mother saying, "Put your napkin in your lap."

When you see your kids doing something right, tell them. When you see them doing something wrong, tell them. **Most of all, your own actions should speak louder than your words.** I'm not sure whether I learned my own values from what my parents said or how they lived their lives. I certainly knew they loved me, but I also knew they expected me to live up to a standard of conduct which was and is not too hard to live up to. Don't be a jerk, be courteous, earn a living, think of others, have decent manners. I remember countless times my mother or father would remind us what appropriate behavior was and what it was not. "When you meet someone, make sure you look them in the eye shake their hand firmly and say their name." I also remember listening to them talk about other families whose parents couldn't or wouldn't teach their kids the rules of life. I think I learned as much from their talking about how not to behave as from the "how to behave lectures." **Why is it that some kids say please and thank you, and some kids don't?**

Help them to make good decisions.

Helping your kids make good decisions requires a lot of making bad decisions — and then learning from them. There is no better teacher than experience. Sometimes we have to screw up in order to go through the kind of emotional experience we need to help us get the message. One of those oft-repeated phrases of my father's was, **"Learning will only take place as a result of an emotional experience."** Quite frankly, I did not get it until I was well into my twenties. It's interesting that my work with people now is to try to create a significant emotional event as a means for people to learn.

My Dad let me make tons of stupid decisions, but he always talked about the stupidity without making me feel like an idiot. Granted, sometimes the price would be too high, so lengthy lecturing was required to prevent my making the mistake. Explaining to your kids the risks of drinking and driving will not guarantee their safety, but we have to do it anyway. That's one lesson that they need not learn from experience alone.

The decision-making process of our brain evolves as we mature, but the more we hang out with our kids and understand them, the more we can help them figure out the best thing to do. Recently, a good friend helped his one son and daughter-in-law with the decision to buy their first home. He explained to him and his new wife that it would be fiscally irresponsible to do that right now. He suggested they work on creating a home, not buying a house. They were, of course, really deflated, but the next day he got a call from his son saying, "Thanks, Dad. I didn't want to hear it but you were right. I really appreciate having you in my life." There are some things, of course, that we can't do anything about. This is the same kid who had in his bedroom a poster that read, "Jim Carey is God." I think he got rid of it when he got married.

Reinforce good habits.

I spoke about this earlier, but it bears repeating. So many parents bitch and complain about their kids. I think they think it's funny or cute. I know I do it. Kids screw up so often that they are an easy target. **But just as good bosses have mastered the art of catching people doing something right, good parents do too.** Go to any Little League game of soccer, baseball or basketball. Just listen to the parents on the sidelines. The coach of our kids' soccer team once handed out a sheet for the parents on how to conduct themselves on the sidelines. It said that we could only yell out positive things to our kids. You could see how the kids responded. It was remarkable how some parents found it too difficult to do — they had to be spoken to. I read somewhere that 85% of parental speech is negative. Like a lot of good habits, the habit of reinforcing good behavior may be hard to learn. Do it anyway. Your kids will notice and remember. And if you have been focusing on their bad habits only, it's never too late to change. Never.

Practice healthy family rituals.

Every family has its own rituals. That's one of the things that makes it your family. **The key is to have rituals that are positive, fun, enriching and "learningful."** They don't necessarily need to be religious, but religious rituals are great for lots of reasons. Going to church or Sunday school as a family is as much about modeling discipline and community involvement as it is about religious training. Having Dad make pancakes on Saturday morning is more than food. It's about Dad connecting with the kids differently. Friday night family movie at home is about togetherness, laughter and learning the moral of the story. Rainy-day board games are about being a gracious winner and loser, and playing by the rules. As kids, we used to have a ritual in the winter after Sunday school. Our whole family would pile into the station wagon and head off to go skiing. We would always eat the tuna fish sandwiches before we even got out of the driveway. It was such a blast. If you think about all the great rituals you currently do, keep doing them. Going to the game, going fishing, cooking together, etc. They have enormous meaning. One family plays "High/Low" at dinner, where they go around the table naming the high point and low point of their day. The game opens the door to real communication about feellngs. Lots of families have bedtime rituals involving stories or songs — rituals that create intimate bonding while getting the kids in the mood to sleep. When I put my kids to bed when they were little, I would always say, **"You're good, you're strong, you're smart, I love you with all my heart."**

The challenge is to knock off the stupid rituals that isolate family members from one another: Eating every meal on the fly. Reading the newspaper while eating. Watching TV while eating. Watching television 8 hours a day. Fighting as a way of communicating. You can think of a few more.

Teach them what you know.

It's not arrogant to say that we as parents know something. We mainly know something because we have lived a little longer and have made more mistakes in our lives. If we have learned a few things about this journey, it's our job to pass it along to our kids so that hopefully their lives can be in some way improved by the wisdom of our years. We don't have all the answers, obviously. But if we can do any good for our kids, it's our duty to try. **Look for teachable moments.**

I could never understand why my father was always talking to me about my life and career, constantly giving advice and counsel. It wasn't that he was a meddling father who couldn't trust his grown son. It was his way of staying connected and being of value. He was constantly giving what he thought was the wisdom of his experience. He was good at doing it in a way that was respectful of my opinion and life. My older sister has many more stories of his advice-giving because he used to come over to their home a lot and dispense wisdom about how to raise the grandchildren. Sometimes it was annoying, but it was also appreciated — not just for the quality of the advice but also because he cared to give it at all. "If you buy a house now, it will nickel and dime you." Or, "If you don't teach her to be nice to people, she will never succeed in life." My sister once wrote a report about who her father was, listing his various accomplishments. He corrected her by saying that his most important role is that of a father.

One time when my sister came home for Thanksgiving vacation from college during her freshman year, she was very sad and told my parents that she no longer felt like part of the family but merely a visitor. This is the letter my Dad wrote to her.

> *Dear Patty,*
>
> *About the visit, and feeling sad or happy or something...Don't think you are alone. We felt sad, too. You know, Patty, it is the nature of thinking people to be sad, <u>sometimes</u>. I am deeply sympathetic. There have been times I have felt thus. (In the army, for example.) There were kids who used to feel sad at camp. Remember? Knowledge helps to temper feeling like this. Also doing things which require knowledge and skill so as to obtain a feeling of accomplishment which comes from a job well done. Dreams are sometimes fun but let us not get too far away from <u>reality</u>. Learn about people and things, and <u>do things,</u> and do them well and this will help to fortify you for those times when things occur which are not completely to your liking. And if you want to know what I'm talking about, I'll come down and we'll talk some day.*
>
> *Love,*
> *Dad*
>
> *P.S. We have nine feet of snow.*

Model honesty, integrity and love.

Kids know a lot more than we give them credit for. **If you live your life in a way that shows them that you're an honest person who has good values and loves them no matter what, I really don't think you can go wrong.** You don't have to be perfect. You can lose your temper, you can make mistakes and you can wonder, "Why did I have kids." Just do your best. Also, make sure you say you're wrong when you're wrong. They appreciate that a lot. If they can't figure out, by the time they've grown, that you're just trying to raise them the best you can, then hopefully another 10 years or so will do the job. The more selfless you can be the better. **The more you can listen without judgment, the better.** Finally, the more you can keep your sense of humor, the better. My mother used to say that we were either hungry or cold whenever we were cranky. Her solution was always, eat something or put on a sweater. My Father would then follow with: "Eat a sweater."

> The other day Jeremy told us that he didn't want to be on the basketball team. He had been to one practice, so we said fine, as long as he called the coach and told him. We explained that it was his responsibility to let the coach know. After several hours of lengthy explanations and crying late into the night, he finally called and left a message on the coach's answering machine saying that he didn't

want to be on the team. We felt proud of him and proud of ourselves. When the coach called back the next day to say that he got Jeremy's message, Jeremy said, "I never said I wanted to be off the team."

If your kids do turn out great, it has something to do with you, but also a lot to do with tons of things you can't control. The same is true if they turn out less than great. Remember that. **Everything a parent does to keep their kids safe can't prevent them from getting sick.** Oh, and one more thing: as Churchill said, never, never, never give up on them.

As far as raising kids goes, there are things that work at some ages that don't work at other ages. There are things that work at some times and not at others. Finally, there are things that work with some kids and never work with other kids. My sister used to call me to ask advice about her three kids at different stages. I think she thought that because I was a trained professional, my counsel would be helpful. Sometimes it was and sometimes it wasn't. The main advice I gave her and parents of kids of all ages, and that we try to follow ourselves, is: **Do what works**. That also means keep trying until you figure out what works. Ask for help if you need to, but remember, **nobody** is an expert with each unique kid.

Having said that, here are some things to avoid because they never work with any kids. They might all fit under the heading, **"What Was I Thinking?"**

Avoid wasting logic.

Using logic with a kid who has crossed into the land of the over-tired or really hungry is obviously a waste of time and energy. I was once describing to a friend how I was having a difficult time arguing with one of my kids after he had melted down right before bedtime. He reminded me that my first mistake was forgetting that it was way past his bedtime, and any rational brain functioning had long since ceased. This also included my brain. There are times when arguing with a teenager is a complete waste of time. Researchers have shown, empirically, that a teenager's brain does not process information the same way as a more mature individual's. This is why the same parents seem to get incredibly smart in the eyes of kids when they are in their twenties.

Avoid trying to make your kid like what you like.

Kids are obviously influenced by our tastes and choices in people and other things, but if you expect your kids to like who or what you do, forget it. I remember my parents wanting me to invite this one kid over to play. I remember thinking, "If you like him so much, why don't you play with him." Here I am, 40 years later, saying, "Why don't you invite so and so over."

Avoid guilt tripping.

It's such a tempting strategy to use guilt to control or manipulate kids to get them to do what is "good" for them, but it usually backfires. "Do you really think that is such a good idea? If you want to, I'm not going to stop you." Or, "If you want to look like that, that's up to you." Or, "I really don't care what you decide to do." Or "I just want you to be happy." Or, "Do you think your hair/sweater/scarf/ looks good that way?" They can tell when they are being manipulated. Unfortunately, not every kid is smart enough to tell his or her parents, "I don't appreciate the subtle guilt trip. If you want me to do or not do something, just say it to me straight." Don't guilt your kids out. It never works.

Avoid avoidance.

It is also a very tempting strategy. You hear it with the comment, "I'm sure the kid will grow up fine, just leave him/her alone — it's a stage." **This is a very common parenting strategy of very busy, or very lazy, or very wimpy parents.** The rationale goes something like this: "I'm an important executive, and I don't have enough time in the day to do all that has to be done, and my spouse does most of the childrearing. She is much better at that sort of thing." Bull. This is called abdicating responsibility. Walking into the other room. Hiding behind the job, the paper, the TV, or the computer is just that. It's hiding.

Oh, and I'd like to blow another myth here. **There is no such thing as quality time.** You only get those moments of quality time when you spend an enormous amount of quantity time. You can also avoid your kids by being with them with a group of other people around. This includes your own family. **You can never get to know your kids if you don't spend lots of time**

185

alone with each of them. That does not mean the 10 minutes you drive with them in the car every morning. It also doesn't mean once a year spending a day with them. Kids will grow up without you being around. Then you can blame their faults on all the lousy influences in their life.

I was talking to an executive the other day about how he stayed connected with his kids although they moved about 10 times throughout their childhood. When his son came home from his new high school one day he told his father after several rounds of silence: "It really sucks being in this new school, Dad." The fact that he could be so honest is the good news. The exec went on to tell me that it hasn't been easy but his kids are doing great in college and they are a stronger family for having weathered the adversity of all the moves. He also believes that the kids are more resilient in their own right for having figured out how to cope in unfamiliar territory. I think he underestimates the impact of what really mattered. He and his wife spent time with them. A lot of time.

Avoid abuse.

Abuse may not be as tempting or as popular as guilt or avoidance, but it is still used by plenty of parents, and it still doesn't work. The abuse I'm talking about here is not physical abuse. If some people reading this book are in the habit of hitting their kids, there is, unfortunately, nothing I can say that will stop them. They are already so steeped in their own stupidity that no argument is going to penetrate. I'm talking about the parents who mentally abuse, embarrass, humiliate, and make their kids feel like failures before they even have a chance at life. Every parent loses his or her temper at times. **The point is that parents can do damage to kids when they let their temper fly out of their mouths with nasty and hurtful things.** I know I've done it, and it never works. Never. I can only hope that my kids are resilient enough and smart enough to know that Dad was acting like a jerk when he said those things, and not internalize them. Have you ever been a spectator at a soccer game and seen what goes on with some parents on the sidelines? Just look at one of those jerks and say, "There but for the grace of God go I." My hope is that the occasions when I do lose my cool with my kids are few and far between. And when I do, I hope I have the humility to say I'm sorry I was wrong. No buts.

The last thing I want to say about kids is to enjoy them at every stage.

There is a glorious sweetness to every stage. Sure, there is also the toxic, rancid and disgusting aspect of every stage, but your job as parents is to focus on the sweet side of your kids' life. I thought it was such a trip how people would react to our twin babies as we strolled through a mall. "Double trouble." Or, "They're sweet now just wait until they become teenagers." I would always say to my wife how their comments were a reflection of their own lives. When my kids were born I felt as though my chest cavity could not contain the love I felt for these two little beings. I remember asking parents of grown children if the love stays as strong as they grow up. They would answer, "Yes, but it changes." The other evening I was staring at one of my boys over dinner, just looking at him and loving and appreciating him for being. It was just my wife and I and one of my boys. I now know why my Dad would stare at me for no apparent reason.

> *Years ago I worked with a family of an adolescent boy who was having all kinds of trouble. He was getting into fights, had lousy grades, and was doing drugs. His relationship with his parents was horrible. But, over many years his parents never gave up on him or each other. Recently, I was privileged to witness one of the most moving wedding ceremonies I have ever seen. This boy survived a non-malignant brain tumor, graduated from college with honors, and became truly a gifted artist. He asked his father to perform the wedding ceremony with his new bride. Many of us in the audience knew what this family had gone through. The love, respect and courage in this family were stronger than any force that might have destroyed them. I don't usually cry at weddings. This one did me in. They are an inspiration to me.*

Parents

The Ten Commandments had it right again. Honor thy father and mother. And your in-laws, too. I know this one is obvious, but there are a few things the Ten

Commandments didn't go into that are useful to remember.

Don't try to change them.

Your mother and father are not perfect. What that means is you cannot expect them to be people that they will never be. Just as with you and your spouse — stop trying to change them. They are not going to change. They are doing the best they can with the resources they have. **If they don't fit your image of what parents should be, grow up!** They don't have to! Expecting them to conform to your idea is your problem. (If I'm starting to sound like Dr. Laura, please shoot me.) It's easy for me to say because my parents were quite normal — and Jan's parents are, too. I know some parents who are fairly nuts, but that is not going to change.

Stay connected.

There are certain things everyone should remember when it comes to dealing with one's parents. Besides not trying to change them, it's also important to stay appropriately connected with them. By appropriately, I mean the right amount of time. For some people, that is a phone call once a week. For others it means having them over for Sunday dinner. My one sister used to talk to my mom every day on the phone. That would drive me nuts. For her, it seemed to work. She was 53 years old and still asked our mom what dress she should wear. I think it was their bonding thing. My Dad and I used to talk about money and work, and they'd talk about clothes and kids. My sister's best friend asked her what she was going to do when my Mom passed away, since she would have no one to dress her. My sister replied, "It wouldn't matter, since no one really cares what I wear except my Mom." **Whatever works for you and your family is what you should do.** Stay connected.

Set boundaries.

Set boundaries that work for you. I can't remember how many families I counseled around the simple act of setting boundaries. I can tell you that not seeing my parents for long stretches of time was both healthy and unhealthy. I certainly appreciated them more when I saw them. On the other hand, they missed out on their grandchildren's lives, and there is even more of a feeling of all of our lives hurtling by. **Make time to connect with your parents and tell them everything you need to before you get that weird phone call in the middle of the night.** Do it now.

Avoid conversational minefields.

Another tip when it comes to parents: Know what to talk about and what not to talk about. This is also related to the skill of setting good boundaries and avoiding pointless and draining arguments. Whether the topic is politics, the proper way to discipline kids, home repairs, relatives, or other juicy issues — they vary, of course, from family to family — you should be smart enough to know when you are likely to be walking into a minefield with only one outcome. I must confess that I sometimes used to enjoy pulling my parents' cork by just mentioning certain people and sitting back to watch the fireworks.

It's a nasty sport. **The bottom line is to exercise some discrimination and some respect with your elders.**

Build and maintain bridges.

Whenever you have a family visit with your parents, keep in mind that you are doing it for a very specific reason. You are building and reinforcing bridges that have stood for decades. Those bridges need to be maintained. A friend of mine spent some time reconnecting with his 80-year-old father. Growing up, he was pretty estranged from his Dad, but in the last few years they've started to spend time talking about things they never talked about. His father told him about his life as a little boy and his experience in the war. He told about meeting his mother, getting divorced, finding love again, and being a parent. Finally, amidst a great deal of seldom-witnessed tears, he shared with his son what it was like to be losing the love of his life. His partner for the last 20 years was dying. My friend did something that I think is very wise. He interviewed his father on videotape. **If it's not too late, interview your parents on tape.** Now.

191

Secrets of the Obvious

- Don't take your marriage or family for granted

- Keep your family boundaries healthy

- Teach your kids your values by living them

- Practice healthy family rituals and traditions

- Avoid toxic behavior with anyone in your family

- Make peace with all your family members, alive or dead

Chapter 9

Financial Health

> *Paul retired from his company after 30
> years. When he walked away he did so
> with a little over 2 million dollars in the
> bank and a healthy pension for life. Over
> those many years he raised three
> daughters, paying for private schools,
> colleges, graduate schools and weddings.
> What Paul lacked in status in his company
> was matched by the financial security that
> he had amassed working, saving and
> investing during this time. He's only 55
> years old and has no financial worries.
> None! Zip, zero, nada. At this point he has
> the luxury of figuring out what to do with
> the second half of his life. His freedom
> from financial stress is not an accident. He
> planned for it with boring dedication. We
> could all learn to be a little more boring.*

There are so many articles, books, magazines, Web sites
and talk shows dealing with money and money
management that it feels somewhat daunting to write a
chapter about the subject. We derive our attitudes about
money not just from these so-called experts, but from
our parents, our friends and our society through its mass
media. Unfortunately, much of what we have been told
and shown is basically untrue. Or more likely, many
important issues weren't discussed at all.

The simple point of this chapter is the following: There are laws of money just like the laws in the other six areas of life. If we ignore these laws, we pay a price (no pun intended). **Fiscal health is about preparation and prevention.** Having money in the bank to weather a fiscal storm is no accident. Nor is it good luck. Stephen Covey is fond of saying that a farmer can't cram for the harvest. If he hasn't done the necessary preparation in the spring, there is no way to harvest in the fall. Get-rich-quick schemes and other strategies are as effective as quick strategies to get friends, lose weight, or produce a great kid. Some of this stuff is so obvious, it seems amazing to me that we forget it and do just the opposite.

Saving

I remember many little aphorisms about money that my Dad told me. One of his favorite lines was, "Put a rubber band around it." This one is a cousin of one of his other favorite lines, "Don't spend." **One of the most basic laws of money is that if you always save at least 10% of your income, you will always live within your means and always have money in the bank.** Paul did that for 30 years.

Everyone already knows that the basic thing that any financial planner will tell you is to pay yourself first. If you don't pay yourself the 10% and put it in the bank, you'll find a way to spend it. People have the capacity to spend whatever they earn. The economist Veblen described the law of "conspicuous consumption." It basically states that our consumption of stuff will increase proportionately to our income. Keeping up with the Joneses is not the only issue. It's that as we make more money we say to ourselves, "I can afford that now." "I deserve that." "I have worked hard." "I've always wanted one of those." This law is like gravity, pulling at us all the time. It is a very powerful force. It occurs inside of us, but it is exploited by the marketing experts who are constantly figuring out ways to suck money from us while making us feel like we're getting a great deal. No money down. No payments for two years. The biggest sale of the year! For a limited time only! Clearance prices! It's not that we shouldn't take advantage of a good deal: It's that we need to be incredibly disciplined about what we can **really** afford.

Banks and credit card companies start soliciting kids when they are 18 years old with offers of credit that they have no business having. What we should teach kids at a very early age is how important it is to save some of what they earn. **If they don't learn it early, it's hard to learn it later.**

I know and you know people who are totally inept when it comes to managing money. It's hard to see our own dysfunction and stupidity when it comes to money, but of course it's easier to see it in someone else. Here are a few beauties that you've probably heard or said:

- *"But I got it on sale"*
- *"I haven't been lucky in the market"*
- *"I'll just charge it"*
- *"I have no idea how much we spend a month"*
- *"As long as I can pay my bills I'm fine"*

- *"I'll worry about retirement later"*
- *"I'll just have to earn more"*
- *"I don't think about money — that's my husband's job"*
- *"I don't need a lot of money to live"*
- *"One of these days I'll be out of debt"*
- *"I know I should watch what I spend but it's too hard"*
- *"The kids wanted it"*

A friend of mine is married and has two kids. He is 46 years old. He pays his bills on time; has a credit card balance that he doesn't pay off every month. He has not saved for the kids' college tuition. He has virtually no retirement savings. He has about $10,000 in the bank. What is wrong with this picture? Luckily for him, if a crisis hits this family, his wife's parents will bail him out. This is no way to live.

Waste and Value

Bert Whitehead is a financial planner whose excellent book *Facing Financial Dysfunction* details some great principles about money. One of the things he talks about is teaching toddlers at an early age **that money is not for eating**. The principle he's referring to is that we shouldn't waste money. Even though my father must have told me a million times to put a rubber band around it, it amazes me how I waste money. Granted, I don't eat it, but I certainly spend money on stuff that is unnecessary and expensive. Sometimes it's because I didn't realize what a waste it was. That's called unconscious incompetence.

A few years ago I bought a Nordic Trak cross country ski machine from my neighbor in a garage sale. It was such a great deal at $100! I never used it for two years and wound up selling it in our own garage sale for $50. It still had the $100 tag on it.

Sometimes it's because I don't take the time to think things through. I recently leased a new car that is quite expensive. The reason I did it was basically because I was too lazy to do the research to find a more appropriate car for my budget. On the other hand, I did a very smart thing with Jan's car. I researched it carefully, and got a great deal on a one year old minivan. Notice how smart I am at economizing when it comes to Jan's car. I know some of you are thinking that getting my wife a used minivan while I cruise in style is somewhat selfish. Actually, Jan couldn't care less about cars. She's as happy as a clam in her minivan.

Everyone knows that if you research a vacation properly and make plans in advance, you can save a lot of money. By the same token, impulse buying, poor planning, and no research are like throwing money in the toilet. I recently re-financed my mortgage and got a significantly lower rate that will save us thousands of dollars in interest payments. The rule we should all follow around big purchases is this: "Wait, let's think this thing through. What is the best use of my time and money? What can we afford? What do we need? What will benefit us the most? Whom should I consult with?" There is a great book by Thomas Stanley and William Danko that many people have read entitled, *The Millionaire Next Door*. The philosophy of this book is very simple: **Don't spend money on frivolous stuff that you don't need.** Look for deals. Live simply. Don't try to impress the neighbors. Be a careful steward to the money you have worked hard to earn.

Let me make something very clear here: **You can also make yourself and everyone around you nuts with an obsession on not wasting a penny.** Clipping coupons and driving around looking for cheap gas can cross the line into penny wise and pound foolish. Not only is it incredibly annoying to hear someone talk about how expensive such and such was, or how you saved 3 cents a gallon on gasoline, it's wasteful in a different way. I know people who will waste time and emotional energy to save a buck. I've done this. I remember going to a fancy restaurant with Jan to celebrate something, but all I could do was comment on how expensive everything was. I ruined the evening for both of us. Haven't we all been in the presence of people whose obsession with how much stuff costs kills the time together?

Value is in the eye of the beholder. How much something is worth has two components. The first is what the thing is worth according to the marketplace. The second is what the thing is worth to us emotionally and personally. Whether some purchase is wasteful or not is both financial and personal. Cars, houses and boats are easy targets for the waste rap. I'm not into boats, but lots of people derive great joy from spending time on their boat, futzing around on the boat, and thinking about how next summer they are going to buy a bigger boat. I could say that such a purchase is wasteful, but that's not my call. If the person can afford it, pays a good price for it, and gets great personal joy from all the things the boat provides, that is hardly wasteful. On the other hand, if the boat sucks money, time and energy from his bank account and his life, I would say it's a waste. And, of course, it's not just boats. It could be antiques, or clothes, or fine restaurants. **If the personal value to you is high and if you can afford the sacrifices you make to get that kind of enjoyment — then go for it!**

My Dad was fond of reminding me how much money a home costs to maintain. He was always cautioning me about buying more than I could afford. When I bought my first home, which was quite old and required a lot of work, he said to me, "If you buy this house you will always hear the voice of the house whispering in your ear, 'Spend money on me. Spend money on me. Spend money on me.'" He was right, of course, and I did sell it after 10 years of decent appreciation and a lot of money spent updating and remodeling.

When I look back on the experience of living in that house, there is no question that Jan and I got a tremendous amount of joy from living there. We remodeled it at least four separate times, but we also had fun doing it. I must say that I love the home we're in now. Granted, it's expensive, but the feeling of joy and serenity I derive from the beauty of the space far outweighs the "expensive" factor. The voice now says,

"Buy me furniture." We're smart enough now to buy furniture that we can afford very slowly. **Decide what is important to you, and spend your money on that.**

Investing

The most important principle to remember is to hire a financial planner if you don't feel completely competent to manage your money. Having said that, I know that people won't do it because they either don't trust anyone to advise them, or they think they can't afford one, or they are too lazy. The reason I recommend a financial planner to help you with your money is because that's what they do for a living. Just like you should go to a doctor for regular checkups, you should go to person who is ethical, competent and willing to help you in your unique situation. I certainly can't recommend an appropriate asset allocation for you, but they can. I have learned so much about money from Bert over the years, but equally important to me is the security and peace of mind I have knowing that there is someone to protect me from my own bad money habits. **All of us have some bad habits when it comes to money.**

When I was in graduate school, I went to a broker who seemed like a nice fellow. He was actually quite new in his profession. I could talk to him easily and we, or should I say I, bought a few stocks on his recommendation. As they started to go down I remember him saying, "If we can just get a bump in the market, I think we'll be OK." Of course, "we" didn't get "a bump" and I suggested we sell. He didn't care, since he made a commission anyway. It was a classic case of the blind leading the blind. The only difference was that he made money and I lost money. I felt like I was in Las Vegas.

Since then, I have read enough investment books to understand the very basics of investing, nothing more. What I have learned from these investment books and magazines, as well as from Bert, are the following simple, obvious laws of investing. These recommendations are **not** about getting rich. This is about having a full tank of gas, a stocked pantry, and a good night's sleep.

- Make sure you have enough liquid cash to allow you and your family to pay all bills for three to six months if you lost your job. Calculate how much that is. Keep that amount in the bank.

- Have an emergency cash reserve equal to 20% of your outstanding mortgage. This is just in case of some serious emergency like losing your job and having some other major crisis. Put this pile in savings bonds or some equivalent interest-earning vehicle.

- Make certain that your investment portfolio is diversified. That means you should never have all of your eggs in one basket — one stock or one asset class. The reasons for this are obvious.

- Fully fund your retirement accounts every year without exception, and watch them grow tax deferred until retirement. Do not touch them until you absolutely have to. **The miracle of compound interest means that time is**

201

worth *more* than money. If you start saving sooner, you'll be wealthier later.

- Establish a long-term investment perspective, but do not walk away from your investment portfolio and allow the "professionals" to manage it. If you smell a lousy decision, or if your goals or risk tolerance change, do something about it. **Do not be passive about your pile.**

The key to investment success is to do what wise, experienced and conservative investors do. They make choices on things they have carefully researched. They don't look to make a quick buck. They understand that the tortoise will beat the hare in the long run. They also know that much of what is hyped in financial publications is bunk. "The top ten stock picks now!" "The best mutual funds to invest in!" "How to guarantee a 20% return!" Read these at your peril and remember that the pills that "melt fat while you sleep!" are sold to suckers every day. Anyone who tells you that they have mastered the market, or their system is fool proof, is a fool. **A fool and his money are soon parted.**

Debt

There are a few facts about debt that you already know. First of all, debt is a pain. Have you ever noticed how great you feel when you pay someone off? Or make that last car payment? Free at last!

There are two kinds of debt: good and bad. Good debt includes home loans, school loans and business loans. This kind of debt uses the power of leverage to allow you to invest in something that should and usually does appreciate over time. Your home, your career and your business should be worth more with time. **Taking out a loan to obtain the degree that you need to further your career is a good debt.** The fact that the government allows you to deduct the interest on your home is another reason to take on this kind of debt. But it is extremely important, even with good debt, not to take on more than you can deal with emotionally and financially. Banks will loan you up to 90% of the value of a home, but conservatively, you should only borrow 50% to 80%. Know what you can handle, not what you are allowed. (If you are not sure about how these two are different, only think of a teenager with a credit card.) Borrowing money to go to medical school is a great reason to go into debt, but even that debt can be an excessive burden. Don't be stupid, even when it comes to good debt.

Now when it comes to bad debt, there is no excuse. **Bad debt includes almost every other kind of debt: long term car loans, consumer loans, and the most disgusting of all, credit card debt.** This is borrowing money on things that will absolutely depreciate in value. Obviously there are times when you have to take out a car loan or finance a large consumer purchase, and there are times when auto companies, for example, offer loans at zero or extremely low interest rates. That's different. The problem is that too many of us forget that credit card debt is really a complete ripoff. **Paying the minimum on a credit card bill is like throwing money away.** But, it's really worse than that. It really lulls us into a false sense of what we think we can afford, and we wind up living beyond our means because we really don't know what we're spending.

Credit card companies basically take advantage of our stupidity, lack of impulse control, and insatiable desire for more stuff. You would need 71 months to pay off a credit card balance of $500 if you made the minimum payment at 14% interest. You would also pay about $200 in interest. That assumes you don't spend another dime during that 71 months. **Decide now that you will never pay a dime of finance charges ever again.** Even if you do, you will become the exception rather the rule.

> *A college student found himself caught by surprise with a tuition bill that he thought his grandmother was going to pay. But she only wanted to pay for 4 years of college, and this was his 5th year. What did he do? He put it on is VISA card, and for 3 years he made the minimum payments. It was only when he went over the limit and VISA threatened legal action that he went to a financial counselor who helped him come up with a more sensible way to manage his debt. In his inexperience, he should have known to get a student loan in the first place. It was too much hassle, and he didn't know how to apply for one.*

Buying Smart: The Law of Tuna Fish and Toilet Paper

The first cousin to avoiding waste is buying smart. The most expensive money you can spend is after tax dollars. You've worked really hard for the money you take home. The government takes its share and then you're left with the rest. We need food, clothing, shelter and a zillion other things to satisfy our need for a decent life in this culture. Andrew Tobias wrote a great book about money entitled *The Only Investment Guide You'll Ever Need.* He made lots of great points, and one that I think is so basic everyone can apply it is the law of tuna fish and toilet paper. He didn't call it that but I like it. He suggested that the easiest way to guarantee that you make 30% on your money is to buy in bulk and wholesale the staples that won't go bad. **If you buy things that you truly need at a 30% discount, your money goes 30% farther.** It's like earning 30% on your hard-earned bread. Go to Sam's Club, Costco, or the equivalent and buy stuff that will not go bad and that you will absolutely use. Of course, if you wind up buying 60 cases of canned smoked oysters that sit in your basement until the kids graduate from college, then that is waste. And if you don't have anywhere to store those rolls of toilet paper, then you probably need to be more selective in your bulk buying.

Getting a great deal on stuff is just smart living. As I said earlier, you don't want to become a nut case or become obnoxious, but you do want to pay less for something if it's possible.

205

> *I had to stay overnight in a hotel at the Detroit airport one evening because my plane got in late and I had to fly out early the next morning. I went to the front desk and asked what the cheapest rate was. The woman said $169. I asked if that was the best she could do. She said, "How about $89?"*

It amazes me how often I've been traveling, and just by asking if I can get a lower rate I usually get one. From hotel room upgrades to cheaper seats on the same plane, it's the same drill. "Do you have one cheaper?" "No" "Are you absolutely certain?" "Well, there is one available." "Thank you, I'll take it." I was surfing the net prior to a family trip and found a great deal at a hotel in Chicago. I called the hotel and asked for the rate. They said they had no such rate. I told them that the rate was available online. They informed me that only if I booked it online could I get the rate. I said OK.

> *A family emergency caused a friend of mine to delay a business trip two days. He had purchased his airline tickets in advance for $277, and when he called the airline, they told him that his new ticket would cost $1200. Later that day he called the same airline, talked with someone else, and found he could use the same ticket with only a $100 penalty.*

People don't ask for a cheaper price because they feel that the printed price must be the price. Or they feel it's impolite to ask for a deal. This is especially true in America, while in other cultures people are insulted if you don't bargain for a lower price. Most car dealers, with a few exceptions, expect you to negotiate and they have some slack built into the list price. And unless the market is exceptionally tight, you can expect to negotiate when you buy a new home. Don't try it with the state trooper who is giving you a speeding ticket, and it probably won't work at the supermarket. But you'd be surprised how often you can get a lower price, especially if you are courteous and respectful when you ask. Enjoy the process.

Some people are too lazy to do the work, or they may lack the confidence. Granted, time is money and you may not have the time to do the research. If you don't have time and it's a major purchase, my suggestion is to get someone to do it for you and pay them; it could be well worth it. Of course, sometimes those cheap airline tickets come with non-financial costs — you may be flying the red eye that lands at 4 a.m. Again, weigh the financial savings against the personal costs.

Speculation

Speculation is not investing. It is the high-risk use of your money with the hope of high return. If you have saved enough money to warrant speculative investments, there are a few things you should remember. You should consider money used for speculative investments to be money you can afford to completely kiss goodbye. **It should amount to no more than 10% of your pile after you have fully funded your retirement**

accounts, your liquid cash reserves, and your emergency cash reserves. Then you can go to Las Vegas, buy lottery tickets and engage in my favorite bad money habit, buying stock on hot stock tips.

I must admit that this is one of the few bad habits that I learned from my Dad. He never knowingly taught me this — he just didn't discourage me from doing it. I suspect he thought it was one of those things like skiing down double black diamond runs: If you can do it and survive, that's great. No guts, no glory. Once again, learning takes place as a result of an emotional experience. I recently decided after thousands of dollars lost in speculative investments to finally listen to my own advice and limit my spec. expenditures to $10,000. The last straw was an investment I made in a company that a guy who cuts my hair told me was a "sure thing." He heard it from someone who heard it from someone who heard it from the horse's mouth. I know this goes in the "what was I thinking" category, but all of us have a story about stupid, hare-brained, risky investments. **The point is that it's OK to take a risk with money you can afford to lose.** Of course, there are some speculative investments that actually do turn out well, and your odds are certainly better than with the lottery. Choose those investments very carefully. And if you enjoy the process — doing the research and watching the market — then have a blast. Just don't play around with the grocery money, your retirement money, or your kids' college money.

Day traders and other gamblers are playing a very risky business. There are plenty of people who think they know something about picking stocks in a bull market. They often forget that a rising tide lifts all boats, or as one entrepreneur said of the dotcom mania, "In a hurricane, even turkeys can fly." When the market makes them look like fools, they'll say they were "unlucky." As my father would say, **"Luck has nothing to do with it."** My friend Ian has been a very successful venture capitalist for over 20 years. It is because he is disciplined, conservative and extremely prudent.

Giving It Away

Now that you've managed to save all this bread, your responsibility is to give it away. There are lots of people who need money and deserve our generosity; the challenge is to give it away properly. You should give it without strings. **You should never give money to anyone or any group and then remind them that you did.** You should also give it without a lot of fanfare. As much as possible you should give it to causes and people that you support but without trying to brag to anyone about how much you gave. My Dad once remarked to me how he found nothing more obnoxious than people who are generous commenting on how generous they are. There is no formula for how much you should give. Some religions recommend giving 10% of your pre- tax income, but I believe that it's up to you and your values. I know people who stopped contributing to the United Fund because the person collecting at work told him what his "fair share" was supposed to be. The act of giving can be enjoyable, and the enjoyment I'm talking about is not in grabbing the spotlight for your generosity. Just make certain the money you donate fits within your budget.

My Dad and Mom were incredibly generous. It wasn't just that they gave a lot of money to causes and people. **It was how they gave.** Whenever they could, they would take the entire extended family on vacations without making anybody feel guilty or beholden. A few summers ago Mom paid for my sisters, her granddaughters, and my wife to go to Europe for a few weeks. She did it out of love and appreciation for them, nothing else. She expected nothing in return and certainly never brought it up. People would say that they would love to be a member of my family or extended family. When people would comment to her on how generous she was, she would look at them in disbelief. In her mind, what else was it for? **Giving away our money is not only for the other people — it's for us.**

Your Money or Your Life

Having a healthy attitude about money is incredibly important in living a healthy and balanced life. There are certain beliefs we hold about money that either help or hinder the way we experience our lives regardless of how much money we make, save, spend, or give away. Making a ton of money or making very little money has nothing to do with whether you live a happy and balanced life — once you get above the starvation level. A researcher once surveyed a wide variety of people at all different economic levels, asking them how much money it would require to make them really happy and secure. The response was consistent:

about twice as much as they had now. This was the case for people earning $250,000 a year and people earning $10,000. Most people think that if they made just a little more money, they'd be happier. Or they think if they had a huge pile of money, they would be really happy.

The truth is that money can make your life a little easier or a lot easier. As a comedian said, "There's one thing money can't buy, and that's poverty." It can give you more choices. It can give you more comfort. It can give you more stuff. It can give you nicer stuff. It can do a lot for you and for others. It is like gas in your tank, or food in your pantry. You can travel farther, or eat better.

What money cannot do is make you happy, fulfilled or challenged. It cannot provide you friendship. As the Beatles said, "Can't Buy Me Love." It cannot get you out of a crummy relationship. It cannot save you from your own delusions. A high school student had both parents die in a car accident, and they left her a large sum of money with no strings attached. The results were predictable: She found herself surrounded by leeches, many of them very unsavory types, and she soon was in jail on drug charges. An extreme example, perhaps, but it makes my point.

I was once asked to contemplate the meaning of the aphorism **"Wealth is a burden to both a rich man and a poor man."** My simple take on that phrase is that to a poor man he thinks of nothing but how he'd like to have more money. He suffers because he thinks that money would solve his problems. The rich man also thinks of money all day and how he can keep all his vast empire safe and sound. What must he do to earn more to keep all the mouths fed, pay the insurance, take the vacations and drive the cars that have become expected? How must he manage the pile of gold?

I don't think a day goes by that I don't think once about money on some level. It's certainly not that I'm poor. Quite the contrary, I think that I sometimes fall into the trap of the successful middle class fellow whose simple appetites have grown as his income has grown. I can hear my Father's comment to me many times, "As much as you earn, you can never earn enough." It wasn't about some arbitrary standard of success. I now understand what he meant. There are always mouths to feed. I think the goal for all of us is to understand that reality and not let it burden you. My sister once asked my Dad whether we were rich. My Dad said to her, "There are some people who have more and some people who have less."

Our responsibility is to earn as much as we are capable or want to while never neglecting or compromising our values or our life. Money is **not** the root of all evil; it is the worship of money that is the root of all evil.

> *My college roommate died from cancer soon after he graduated from Yale Law School. He came from a middle class family on Long Island. His father was in the construction business in New York City. Sitting in the hospital one night, I asked his father about his perspective on life. I*

don't remember what I asked exactly, but to this day I remember very vividly something he said. He was sad about his son, but he was more upset about the dark side of human nature. "Oh, Harry, you would not believe what I have seen over the years — how people will do anything for the holy buck. It's enough to make you sick."

We should treat money with great reverence without worshiping it. It is not always easy to do. Just like teaching toddlers not to eat it, we should respect money and use it properly as a fuel that allows us to move through life with ease. A colleague of mine, a talented and successful management consultant running her own business, told me that she has some really stupid deep-seated beliefs about money that keep her from being more successful. Something along the lines of thinking that it's not OK to make lots of money. As a result, she frequently under-charges for her time and services. We live in a society in which people pay for what they value. If she values the contribution she makes, she will charge more for her services. If people value those services, they will pay for them. I don't think she is alone in her misconceptions about money. We all have work to do.

I'd like to think that the values Jan and I are teaching our kids about money will serve them well in their lives. Beyond the "money doesn't grow on trees" stuff, I think the understanding of money is a lifelong challenge. I not only care that they can earn a decent living and support their families and communities, but that they have the right perspective about money. I have seen in therapy a lot of people who were never taught the proper value of money in one's life. I'm still working on it.

Secrets of the Obvious

- Save at least 10% of your income, and make that saving as painlessly automatic as possible

- Have a financial plan

- Do some homework. Buy smart. Ask for deals

- Spend money on what is important to you

- Research and monitor your investment choices, and don't invest to get rich quick

- Give your money away in ways that enrich your life and others

Chapter 10

Spiritual Health

Greg and I were out after a movie last Friday night, and he shared with me what it has been like living with his wife for the last few years. It has been so painful for him to watch her slowly deteriorating health and loss of mind that he often hides his sadness about her condition because he is afraid of bumming her out. He has no one with whom to share his anger and sadness but his close friends, but even we can't really feel what it's like to live with and love a person in chronic pain and no diagnosis that gives any hope. What he shared the other night was something he never revealed to anyone. Through a great deal of meditation and prayer he has come to see his suffering and the suffering of his wife as a great gift. It has allowed him to feel a level of compassion for others that he never would have experienced without this pain. In his eyes, the gateway to God or any spiritual experience is through our suffering. For that experience he is truly grateful. For the first time in his life he feels that he has found both meaning and peace. More important, it has not been a fleeting glimpse. He has been able to bring that peace to his work with clients and, most important, to his relationship with Linda. It's not about being intellectually clever with esoteric spiritual truths — he's really doing great. There is a lightness to Greg that is wonderful to behold.

Some people get very uncomfortable around the topic of spiritual health because they think it's too personal and private to talk about. Some also have had very mixed experiences with "religious" traditions and the people who were supposed to teach them about those traditions. Obviously, all religious fanaticism is repulsive — because of its bigotry toward anyone who follows a different spiritual path — that it's hard to get past it sometimes to realize the importance of spiritual seeking.

Despite these difficulties, spiritual health may be as important to cultivate as all of the other categories of healthy living combined. Let's face it, when you're trapped under a building, or on your own death bed, or watching hopelessly as a loved one suffers, or dealing with the meaning of life, this category of health may be the most important. But we don't need to have a catastrophe happen to have our spiritual health provide us with enormous power. There is no single right way to cultivate this area of our lives, but there are very specific things we can do — or not do — that will make a huge difference to our quality of life. **Some things require more effort than other things, but like all of the rest of the seven areas of healthy living, with effort comes grace.** The key is keep searching until you find the right path for you.

Be a Seeker

When I was 18 years old my senior project in high school was to spend a month doing anything I wanted to do that had some educational value. One kid learned to play the banjo. Another worked on a farm. I chose to live in an ashram for a month and study yoga. An ashram is like a monastery. Lots of silence, prayer and meditation. I was raised as a Jew, and part of my own faith was to contemplate the meaning of life. That month was focused on just that. What it taught me is incredibly simple: **Our goal in life is to know God.** Here's the cool part: There are a million ways to do that, of course, and no one faith or practice has the inside track. There are many paths to the summit of the mountain. What I learned in that Ashram was that we are all seekers of the Truth in one way or another. Some people do it in a very deliberate way with scriptures and rules and regulations. Some people do it in their own unique way which other people think is stupid. **Find what works for you, and do that.** You don't even have to use the word God. Every faith and religious tradition has the same goal nonetheless.

My wife and I recently started to send our kids to Sunday school to help them to understand their faith more than they currently do. Jan and I started to attend a Torah study with the Rabbi while the kids were in class. What amazed both of us was not that the experience was fabulous. It wasn't really. What was great about the experience was how we finally understood the meaning behind practices and rituals we had been doing all our lives. In fact, one of the things that we discussed last

217

week is that unless one understands the point of any spiritual practice or ritual, it becomes empty and meaningless. **The purpose of prayer is to make the one who is praying become a better person after having prayed.** It's not to get what one is praying for. The point is simply to make the effort to put yourself in a position of humility. The Ten Commandments are about how to live in this world as a moral and ethical person with commitment to God, family and society at all times.

I never quite got the notion of "Remember the Sabbath day and keep it holy." The deeper meaning behind that commandment is to stop and take stock, to pause in our rushing, and to give thanks. And you don't have to wait until the weekend! People who study scripture much more diligently than I do are always quoting a passage from the Bible that informs their lives in a real way. That's the whole point. The manager who retired with $2 million recently told me that he and his wife believe in a proverb that made their lives easier, "Honor the Lord with your wealth, with the first fruits of all your crops; then your barns will be filled to overflowing and your vats will brim over with new wine."

The study and practice of any religion or spiritual path is not to become holier than thou, it is to make yourself a better person as you live your daily life. It's to make sense out of this mundane world so you are uplifted and uplifting. Greg's spiritual insight about the importance of suffering as a means of cultivating our compassion is about having that compassion in the midst of our daily lives with ourselves and strangers, not just with our suffering loved ones.

My thirteen-year-old niece, Lauren, recently completed her Bat Mitzvah. This ancient Jewish ritual of coming-of-age had more significance than any I have ever attended. One year previously this young girl had been hospitalized with anorexia. In the year she recovered from the brink of death, her parents, grandparents, friends and doctors never gave up on her. The scripture she read at her Bat Mitzvah had incredible meaning to those of us who knew what she had overcome. She described the biblical story of King Saul, his son, Jonathan, and Jonathan's friend, David. Saul was plotting to kill David and asked his son, Jonathan, to lure David to his death. Out of loyalty to his friend, Jonathan warned David and saved his life. Lauren talked about what the story meant to her in terms of courage, friendship and loyalty, and concluded her talk with a reminder that all of us have been — or are — a "Jonathan" to someone, and someone is a "Jonathan" to us. She shared that she wouldn't be alive today were it not for the family and friends who stood by her like Jonathan. All of us knew just what she meant.

As I was telling my friend Bob about this chapter he reminded me that it is important to clarify that being a seeker is not about going to formal places of worship. Rather, it is about seeking the sense of spirituality or meaning or purpose in everyday life. He suggested that I talk about tools that help people do just that. For example, the practice of gratitude is a spiritual practice. **The deeper challenge for all of us is not just to feel gratitude for situations but gratitude in situations.**

My sister has cancer right now and is going through chemotherapy. This woman is a model of gratitude. When she first found out, her attitude was so positive about how great her life had been up until this point. It's not that she wanted to die, but she was so at peace with what was happening to her. She figured that she would do whatever was necessary, but then if it was her time, then it was her time — so be it. She is sending the coolest e-mails to all her friends and family about how great it is to have cancer. People shower her with food and attention, they express their love, affection and appreciation, and she gets to reflect on the meaning of life. Her sense of humor is still intact even though she feels awful and has no hair. She sends out these great weekly updates about what she's going through. In fact, the Roswell Park Cancer Institute asked her to collect these e-mails into a book entitled "Humor after the Tumor." This is one e-mail she sent out recently. (Kambel is their golden retriever.)

> *I feel so good that I am wondering if they forgot to put the Taxol in my drip! The warmer weather has felt great too. I've been walking around the neighborhood with the dogs and without my hair; not only does it feel more comfortable but also I am convinced that sunshine will help my hair grow! It works for grass! One pleasing side effect of the last drug was the loss of my facial hair; let's hope that the inch which Sharon promised does not grow in as a mustache instead of a brush cut! Another reason I don't wear the*

*wig most of the time is because it's hot! It
washes easily, but I have to be careful
where I hang it to dry. I found Kambel
running through the house with it, so
excited. I really couldn't blame him; when
it hangs on a doorknob or lies on a
counter it looks like a squirrel!*

Enjoy and feel as good as I do!

*Love,
Patty*

Patty has always had this great attitude about life. She
doesn't think about life after death. She thinks about her
life before her death. She is a great example of gratitude
and grace under pressure. Her attitude is that you should
not burden people with your suffering; you should make
it as easy as possible on them. Her sense of humor isn't
a cover up for her pain. When she is hurting, she has no
trouble telling you what's going on in great detail, but
she knows that what's important is not how she's feeling
but how she makes others feel. I admire her a lot.

**You don't have to get cancer in order to develop a
spiritual perspective, or follow a spiritual Path, or
know God — however you want to describe it.** Yes,
getting cancer or losing a loved one can make us stop in
our tracks, set aside our routines, take stock, and think
about the Big Picture stuff: What am I doing with my
life? What should I be doing? We can all make an effort,
through prayer or meditation, through pauses to think

and feel, or through being mindful of what we are doing in our daily lives. This is what I mean by being a seeker.

Karma and Dharma

If it's one thing I want to teach our kids, it's the law of Karma and the meaning of Dharma. Yes, I was raised as a Jew, but as I said, the right Path for us is the one that leads us towards the Truth. I first learned the concepts of Karma and Dharma from my years of studying yoga, but they have been a profound help to me over the years of doing therapy, corporate consulting, and quite frankly, living my life. You don't have to use the terms to get the point. As I was explaining Karma to one of my sons he said, "You mean what goes around, comes around?" He understood it completely. The law of Karma, as I have understood it, is that whatever we do has an impact on the world. **We are constantly planting seeds, with every single thought, word and deed.** Those seeds will eventually sprout into something or other if the right conditions prevail. Therefore we should, as much as possible, be conscious of what we are sowing. We may not see the fruits of those seeds immediately, and we may not see them ever, but we are planting them nonetheless.

Instant Karma is the easiest to see. When we overeat, we feel sick. Stay up late, wake up tired, rush to work. Smile at a stranger and immediately watch the result. **The longer- germinating seeds are harder to see.** When we accomplish anything, it's not an accident. When something "happens" to us, sometimes, upon reflection,

222

it becomes obvious how we l
Good stuff or bad.

> *When I was in privat*
> *of young teens. M*
> *dealing with drugs*
> *One kid was extreme*
> *quite get how he h*
> *luck" he kept havin*
> *explained to him that if you plant apple seeds, you will get an apple tree and eventually apples will fall from the trees. If you are walking under that tree, an apple may fall on your head. If you plant turd seeds and walk under that tree, the same rules apply. Smoke pot, hang around with losers, you will eventually get busted. He got it.*

To the best of our ability we should plant wonderful things in the fertile soil of our minds. We should monitor the stuff we fill our heads with. This includes the stuff we watch to the stuff we read to the stuff we think. We should plant wonderful things with our words. We've all made stupid mistakes by saying things that we wished we'd not. The ancient Sufi aphorism states, **"Before any words leave your lips may they pass through three gates. May they be <u>truthful</u>, may they be <u>necessary</u>, may they be <u>kind</u>. If they are all three, they may leave your lips."**

Granted, these are hard criteria to live up to, but so what. Remember the implications of your words.

...ctions should be those that we can be proud ...ey will have a consequence — seen or unseen. ...al is to be conscious.** Then we at least have a ...ce to watch how we are tending our garden. Look ...round you; look at what you are creating. It's quite amazing that people who work very hard and treat people very well are often very "lucky."

> There is an old Zen story about a Master walking with his student, when the student stops to tie his shoes because they had become loose. Just then a huge boulder crashes down a hillside and almost crushes both of them. The Master then explains to the student, "We have no control over when that boulder comes crashing down. We have no control over whether our shoes become untied. All we have control over is how well we tie our shoes." There are plenty of shoes in our lives that we have control over.

The meaning of Dharma is a little more complicated to understand. The easiest translation is "righteous duty" but that doesn't do it justice. **To do one's Dharma is to do what is right.** It is not always easy to know or see what is right, but that's the way it is. It really means to contemplate your values and act in accordance with those values. Sometimes it seems that there is no clear answer. That's where the effort comes in. Trying to figure out what path is the most Dharmic is actually a spiritual practice in itself. How can I earn a living and spend time with my family and be a good citizen and take care of my health and . . .? That's what Dharma is all about.

It is our responsibility to figure that out and make choices among all the conflicting demands for our time. In this moment I should be with my kids with complete attention. In the next moment maybe I should be at work with the same attention. The next moment maybe I should be talking to my sister. We all know what it feels like to have made the right choice with our time. Or, for that matter, the wrong choice. **The question that many people ask, "What should I be doing with my life?" is a great question. The answer is, figure it out.** Find what your mission is in life. The smaller decisions are easier when your values are clear.

> *A friend of mine whose wife has Hodgkin's Disease was having a spiritual crisis because he felt guilty leaving his wife alone to travel to Michigan to work all week and then fly home to Tennessee on Thursday. She helped him enormously without saying, "Jon this is your Dharma." She just told him that the right place for him was doing what he loves and needs to do to support his family. He is a gifted facilitator and should be working. She also knows that if she needs him, his Dharma is to be back at home with her. There was a time recently when he had to leave work and be with her. There is a profound*

simplicity and peace when we are clear
about what is the right thing to do.

Meditate or Pray

Meditation and prayer are spiritual practices within every religious tradition. **Even if you don't have a religious bent, you can do either or both.** The reasons are the same as the reasons why you should exercise: because it works. In the same way that exercise invigorates the body and the mind, meditation and prayer invigorate an important part of who we are. All of us can exist just fine without exercise, but we function so much better when we do. The same is true for prayer and meditation. The effect is more subtle but no less important. If you meditate regularly or have a life of prayer, you can access a certain degree of peacefulness more easily than if you don't. It's that simple. **The benefit is not just peacefulness; it's also a certain perspective about life.**

When you meditate, you just sit in a comfortable position, listen to your breathing, repeat a phrase if you want to, and just watch what happens. Yes, it's that simple. More often than not you watch millions of thoughts float by. Occasionally you get caught up in the thought, run around for a while, and then come back to your breathing. Don't expect anything to happen — just watch what happens. There comes a moment when you realize that you are the one who is watching without judgment. This Consciousness who is watching some call God or the inner Self or the Witness. It doesn't matter at all what It is called. What you experience is that you are not your thoughts. That is a profound experience in itself. If you hang in there long enough, you seem to disappear completely. It's like you're asleep but not really. You then open your eyes and feel great. The experience also lasts longer than the few seconds after you open your eyes. The realization that you are not your thoughts gives you the same freedom as the marathon runner feels when he knows that the pain in his legs is only temporary and he is not going to be a victim of his discomfort. He knows he is more than his body. As you go through your day you can stop and remember more easily that what is happening to you is a movie playing inside your head. This too shall pass. **You don't have to be victimized by whatever is happening to you.**

Let me be crystal clear. The purpose of meditating or praying is not to reach some altered state of consciousness and become a spiritual person of some sort. You're already a spiritual person. **The point of meditation and prayer is to live your current life with more grace and equanimity.** Who doesn't want that? Well, come to think of it, lots of people, but this book isn't for them anyway.

> *The Zen student asked the Master what one did before enlightenment. The Master replied, "Chop wood and carry water." Then the student asked, "What about after enlightenment?" The Master replied, "Chop wood and carry water."*

Prayer is the same as meditation, only there are a lot more words. Some people have favorite prayers. Other people pray by talking very personally to their unique and private experience of the Divine. **The point of prayer is to place yourself in relationship to Something or Someone greater than yourself.** The very act of prayer invokes a state of humility and gratitude. Whether it means getting on your knees or bowing your head, the symbolism is about getting your head below your heart. **Prayer is about putting yourself in a position of being a servant to something greater than your own desires.** Usually there is a request to make oneself a better person in some way. What could possibly be wrong with that?

These are some of my favorites:

> *O God, keep my tongue from evil and my lips from speaking guile. Be my support when grief silences my voice and my comfort when woe bends my spirit. Plant humility in my soul, and strengthen my heart with perfect faith in Thee. Help me be strong in trial and temptation and to be patient and forgiving when others wrong me. Guide me by the light of Thy counsel, that I may ever find strength in Thee, my Rock and my Redeemer. Amen.* (Union Prayer Book)

> *Lord, make me an instrument of your peace. Where there is hatred let me sow love; Where there is injury, pardon; Where there is doubt, faith; Where there is despair, hope; Where there is darkness,*

light; Where there is sadness, joy. O Divine Master grant that I may not so much seek to be consoled as to console; to be understood as to understand; to be loved as to love. For it is in giving that we receive; it is in pardoning that we are pardoned; and it is in dying that we are born to eternal life. (Saint Francis of Assisi)

God, grant me the serenity to accept the things I cannot change, the courage to change the things I can, and the wisdom to know the difference. (Serenity Prayer)

I will do Thy bidding. (Bhagavad-Gita)

Pray any way you want to. If you like to read scriptures or inspirational writing, do that. Some find it helpful to feel part of an ongoing tradition because you don't feel so alone. Others prefer to pray in their own personal words. The point is to do it with the right attitude. As the rock lyric from the Doors goes, "You cannot petition the Lord with prayer." The image that comes to mind is the gambler watching the roulette wheel while praying fervently, "Please Lord, red 27." **The goal of praying is not to get something but to give something.** With that attitude in mind, you cannot go wrong.

One more thing about meditation or prayer: Keep it to yourself. **Don't go talking about how much you pray or how often.** Don't go talking about how much you meditate or what great experiences you are having. Don't tell people you are reading scripture every day. The more you talk about your private moments of connection to the ineffable, the more you cheapen and sully the experience. You also risk alienating people with your spiritual materialism. There is nothing more obnoxious than people who imply or tell you how spiritual they are. **Just chop wood and carry water.**

I mentioned earlier that it has been said that the two wings of the bird of enlightenment are Grace and Effort. **We are only responsible for the effort; the Grace will be bestowed upon us for reasons that are beyond our comprehension.** What that means is we have the awesome responsibility to put forth effort. Sometimes a lot of effort is required, sometimes a little effort. If our lives don't seem to be working out the way we would like, the answer is simple and obvious: Put in more effort. Don't whine, don't complain, just do what needs to be done without fanfare or flurry. A friend suggested that I write about why people don't do all the things I mentioned in this book. I should go into all of the obstacles of why people don't do what is good for them. The answer is obvious: People are lazy. We don't like to work hard. We would rather complain about what isn't working than change ourselves, our attitudes, our habits, our friends, our work, our lives. **If crops won't grow after all of your watering, fertilizing, and pruning, plant your garden elsewhere.**

Leave a Legacy

A few weeks ago my mom passed away. She was 79 and for many years we in the family had joked about how she would go, since it really was a matter of time. She had breast cancer 20 years ago, but other than being overweight and having high blood pressure, she wasn't in poor health. Her mind was as sharp as a tack. She found out she had lung cancer on Jan. 8. On February 19 she was dead. Earlier in this book I mentioned that it was important to video your parents before it was too late. I thank God I did. I sat down with my sister and my mom and asked her lots of questions about her life and her thoughts about her death. What she told us was truly priceless. I thought I would have many more times to videotape her, but that wasn't in the cards. I will try and convey some of the gems of that one conversation.

She talked about how she wanted the funeral to go and what should be served at the reception. She had gone over with Patty what she wanted read about her, and then as Patty was reading it to her she corrected her by reminding Patty that it was to be about her and Herman. Her happiest days were the 51 years she spent with her best friend, Hermie. She talked about how the important things in life are to be a good person and raise your kids to be happy, productive members of society with a means of taking care of themselves. She talked about how you should treat your family like friends and your friends like family. When I asked her to elaborate, she explained that too many people take their family members for granted and don't treat them as well as their friends, and they don't allow their friends to get close to them like family. She talked about how it was time to go and that you should have no regrets when it's your time, because it's time to make room for the new. She wanted all of us to remember that she had a great life, but it was now time to focus on our lives.

I've watched that tape several times since her death. When I think about how she died and what she told us, I am incredibly grateful for the legacy she left. She modeled for all of us how to live and how to die. My mother was not faking it. That was not her style. She called it exactly as she saw it. What a rock! She wasn't trying to be spiritual. There was no guilt. There was no regret. There was no anger at being taken when there was more to do. It was a straight, "OK, I've had a great life. Now go live yours well." **The legacy she left was to live a life that matters.** Make a difference in the lives of others. She did.

My cousin wrote this letter to my family the day of the funeral.

> I just heard about Millicent. I can only imagine the richness of having had Millicent in your lives for so many years. When Millicent and Herme came by for a brief visit many years ago, I was fortunate to catch a glimpse of who she was. Herme was very proud of her. He beamed as he spoke about how she was with people — strong, assertive, and charming. I could see his appreciation of her and her talents. I spoke to her a couple of weeks ago and told her how important our conversations had always been to me. She was always interested in my life and her perspectives were always on the mark. She had a very special way of reaching people. I never felt

defensive and always valued our talks.
How fortunate you all were to have had
Millicent in your lives. If I felt enriched by
our few brief yearly contacts, I can only
imagine what you felt.

Love,
Susan

Remember what I said earlier about planting seeds. The words that we use and the things that we do, even the little things, have an impact. They become our legacy, our gifts to the world. In some cases they may be summed up, as with my mom's wise words on her video or my father's wise words to me at various times in his life. But even if that doesn't happen, the summation of our lives becomes the legacy we leave behind for others. Make it a good one. **Now.**

Secrets of the Obvious

- Be a seeker

- Do Good: Karma and Dharma

- Meditate or pray

- Live a life that matters

- Leave a legacy

Chapter 11

Obviously, Not the End

In 1927, Max Ehrmann, a poet and lawyer from Terre Haute, Indiana, wrote this in his diary: *"I should like, if I could, to leave a humble gift -- a bit of chaste prose that had caught up some noble moods."*

He then penned a poem – the "humble gift" he was looking for – and called it *Desiderata*, Latin for "things to be desired." Years passed, Mr. Ehrmann passed away, and then, in the late 1950s, the Rev. Frederick Kates, the rector of St. Paul's Church in Baltimore, Maryland, used the nearly forgotten poem in devotional materials he compiled for his congregation.

I present it here in its entirety as a parting gift to you — as poetic a description of balance as any I've found. Enjoy...

235

Desiderata

Go placidly amid the noise and haste
and remember what peace there may be in silence.
As far as possible, without surrender,
be on good terms with all persons.
Speak your truth quietly and clearly; and listen to others,
even the dull and the ignorant; they too have their story.
Avoid loud and aggressive persons; they are vexations to
the spirit. If you compare yourself with others,
you may become vain and bitter; for always there will be
greater and lesser persons than yourself.
Enjoy your achievements as well as your plans.
Keep interested in your own career, however humble; it
is a real possession in the changing fortunes of time.
Exercise caution in your business affairs; for the world is
full of trickery. But let this not blind you to what virtue
there is; many persons strive for high ideals;
and everywhere life is full of heroism.
Be yourself. Especially, do not feign affection.
Neither be cynical about love; for in the face of all aridity
and disenchantment it is perennial as the grass.
Take kindly the counsel of the years, gracefully
surrendering the things of youth. Nurture strength of
spirit to shield you in sudden misfortune. But do not
distress yourself with imaginings. Many fears are born of
fatigue and loneliness. Beyond a wholesome discipline,
be gentle with yourself.
You are a child of the universe, no less than the trees
and the stars; you have a right to be here.
And whether or not it is clear to you the universe is
unfolding as it should. Therefore, be at peace with God,
whatever you conceive Him to be.

236

And whatever your labors and aspirations, in the noisy confusion of life, keep peace with your soul. With all its sham, drudgery and broken dreams, it is still a beautiful world. Be cheerful. Strive to be happy.

Max Ehrmann, 1927

Desiderata (as applied to the Seven areas of healthy living)

Physical: Beyond a wholesome discipline, be gentle with yourself.

Psychological: Nurture strength of spirit to shield you in sudden misfortune. But do not distress yourself with imaginings.

Social: As far as possible without surrender be on good terms with all people.

Work: Keep interested in your own career, however humble, it is a real possession in the changing fortunes of time.

Family: Especially, do not feign affection. Neither be cynical about love; for in the face of all aridity and disenchantment it is as perennial as the grass.

Financial: If you compare yourself to others, you may become vain and bitter; for always there will be greater and lesser persons than yourself.

Spiritual: Therefore, be at peace with God, whatever you conceive Him to be. And whatever your labors and aspirations, in the noisy confusion of life, keep peace with your soul.

Secrets on the Web

Like you, I am ever learning. Fortunately, the Internet and the World Wide Web have made it easier to share that learning on a more timely basis than having to wait for a second or third edition of a book. If you would like to share your "secrets of the obvious" or simply hear what others have to say, visit www.secretsoftheobvious.com. I hope to hear from you soon!

About the Author

Harry Cohen has worked with over 150,000 executives, entrepreneurs, managers and corporate employees throughout North America and Europe. Since 1995 he has been one of the principal developers and lead presenters at Ford Motor Company's Excellence in Leadership Conference for over 3,000 management teams from across the United States and Canada. In addition to conducting hundreds of 3½-day conferences, he has presented via satellite to organizations since 1996.

Harry received his B.A. in psychology from Cornell and his Ph.D. from the University of Michigan. He and his wife, Jan, and their sons Ethan and Jeremy live in Ann Arbor, Michigan.

If you would like to contact Harry, his email address is harrydcohen@comcast.net